YOUR
SELFCARE MATRIX

10 Critical Principles to Effectively Improve Awareness, Communicate Your Needs, and Manage Your Health Naturally

by

DENISE NICHOLS

SELFCARE MATRIX GUIDEBOOK

READ THIS FIRST

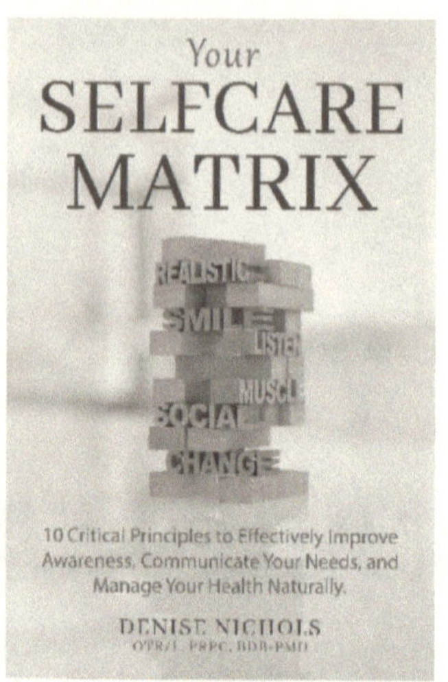

Just to say thanks for buying this book I would like to give you the Guidebook for FREE.

You will be most successful if you use the Guidebook to set your goals and complete the exercises as you read. This is your commitment to embracing change and making healthcare work for you. Starting new habits takes dedication and commitment. Research shows that writing down your goals and plans makes you much more likely to be successful. Take the time to write things down as you go. Making it work for you starts with you.

http://selfcarematrix.com/

"I'm trying to free your mind. But I can only open the door. You're the one that has to walk through it."

— *Morpheus (The Matrix)*

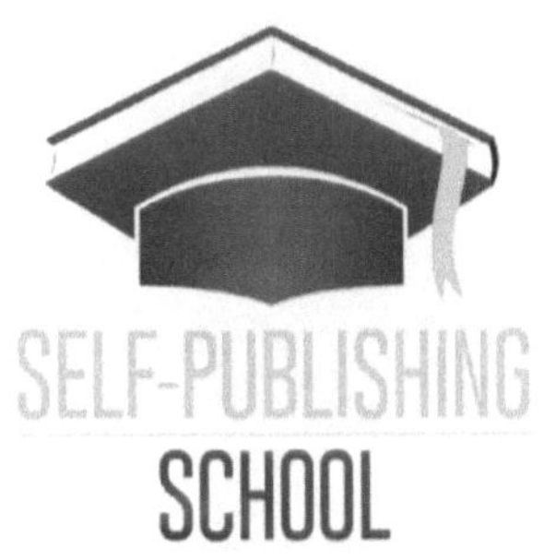

SELF-PUBLISHING
SCHOOL

ISBN: 9781731200174

DEDICATION

This is dedicated first and foremost to my husband Craig, for supporting me through every obstacle and sharing in every joy. He is the rock on which my circle of trust is built. Next, to my children, Mckena and Cadan, as well as my family and friends who have put up with so much yet love me unconditionally. I also dedicate this book to every patient and healthcare member alike. You are all warriors. Keep embracing Change.

"Don't Think Outside the Box. Think Like There is No Box."
— *Motivation Project*

"Self-care has become a new priority – the revelation that it's perfectly permissible to listen to your body and do what it needs."

— *Frances Ryan*

TABLE OF CONTENTS

PRINCIPLE #2: IDENTIFY WHAT'S HOLDING YOU BACK 24

GOALS FOR THE READER

i.   Learn why putting selfcare as the foundation to your healthcare is critical to the success of your health and wellness (and how to achieve it!).

ii.   Learn the new definitions of selfcare and healthcare and how to make them both work for you.

iii.   Learn how to identify and then let go of what is holding you back.

iv.   Learn how to find, build, and navigate a "self-health care" team that acknowledges and respects your selfcare priorities.

v.   Commit to CHANGE and understand how to easily apply these core values every day.

vi.   Learn how to hear and listen to your body's signals.

vii.   Learn how to interpret your body's signals based on educated and informed awareness of how YOUR body works.

viii.   Learn how to effectively communicate and follow through on your ever-changing healthcare needs based on daily awareness.

ix.   Establish and set a flexible plan with realistic goals.

x.   Learn how to balance your "whole" self with the 8 "S" Rule.

ACKNOWLEDGMENTS

I would like to acknowledge those who have supported, and sometimes carried, me every step of the way, through life, Lyme, and the crazy rollercoaster ride titled "Writing a Book."

Craig Nichols
Andrew Kopecky
Pam and Chip Chapdelaine
Lise Cartwright
Christos Angelidakis

I would also like to acknowledge the people who have inspired me to step outside of my comfort zone and really explore who I am and what kind of mark I want to leave on this world before I leave.

Amanda Bush
Erica Hoyer
Shiraz Tata
Chad Madden
Chandler Bolt

And to my amazing Motivate team. They are living proof that you can love what you do and make a difference in this world simply using your passion to help others. I am forever grateful for their support, dedication, and hard work.

Barb Rigsby
Donna Moore
Rinelle Culver
Lisa Edwards
Sharon Fritts
Kait Baer
Shana Schwanebeck

INTRODUCTION

"The most powerful relationship you will ever have is the relationship with yourself."

— *Steve Maraboli*

What the Heck is My Selfcare Matrix?

Your Selfcare Matrix is an organized model built to help guide and support you along your health and wellness journey. The six layers are built from the 10 principles, creating an easy-to-follow guideline that you can use to assess your daily choices and habits, set goals, and communicate your ever-changing healthcare needs.

"Matrix" can be a complicated concept. It is made up of many moving parts, whether we are talking mathematics or the human body. It is a mold from which we build a solid, yet constantly moving structure. I propose that selfcare and healthcare co-exist. You are the selfcare matrix, the environment from which something develops. A matrix is made up of constantly moving parts, and you are the sum of those parts.[7] You are not alone. You need amazing healthcare team members, but there should be no separation between selfcare and healthcare.

The "foundation" of your matrix are the core values

selfcare matrix

of CHANGE from which your selfcare choices should be based upon. These choices come from your improved awareness of how your body works, as represented by the next two layers. Only from that awareness can you effectively communicate your needs and then create REAL goals. Last, but not least, comes putting it all together and learning to live a balanced, high quality of life.

The balancing block game featured on the cover perfectly conveys how, true to matrix form, the pieces are built to move, glide and slide. But if one piece falls out of line, it can affect the balance of the entire structure. In this case, your health and quality of life.

What is Selfcare and Why is it So Important?

Selfcare is dancing, laughing, and crying. It is walking, running, talking, being silent, sitting, exercising and making love, drinking, eating, peeing, pooping, and sleeping. If your mind and body need it, you do it. Basic "self-care" is what we do automatically. When we feel the urge to pee, we go to the bathroom, (at least we are supposed to). The Selfcare Matrix is all about the quality of care that you do for yourself and what you expect from others. This includes your friends, family, and healthcare team.

Closing the door, planting both feet on the ground, breathing, taking your time to use the bathroom—*peeing with awareness!*—instead of peeing while dealing with fighting children. Relaxing, allowing things to happen naturally. Not thinking about what you haven't done or what you need to do, that is self-care.

Taking care of YOU so that you can do everything from the basics of survival to the deep "living life" moments—that is selfcare! It is doing what you love, and often what you don't. It is finding the power within.

That power, or inner fire, has always been there and always will be. But you need to reconnect with it every moment of every day. You have limitless potential; it is who you are.

Self-awareness is the key. It's your inner fire—the power of connecting with yourself and connecting with others. The power to connect with the universe, the "everything" that is "everywhere"—we are all a part of it. It is the ability to see ourselves clearly, to see how others see us, and to see how we fit into the world.[24] The lie that that we live with every day is that we are separate, alone. We are all part of this whole, big, crazy world, and that makes us humans a team—a team of teams. You may not like having to rely on others, but until you see the truth that you need others to help you care for you, you will not be "wholly" healthy, "wholly YOU". That is selfcare.

How Do I Make This Book Work for Me?

This book is your map. The guide that shows you how to prioritize your needs based on your body's basic and more complex signals. It will show you how to build your healthcare team and how to rely on team support from a matrix of selfcare, with you at the center.

The term 'matrix' is a noun and refers to something that begins or develops from within.[25] It is the place from which your healthcare should develop and blossom. You are the foundation of this "self-health care matrix". CHANGE will occur from your awareness. That is how we will fix our currently rather fragmented healthcare system, one person at a time.

What is an Empowered Patient and How Do I Become One?

Pure and simple. It is well-agreed that knowledge is power. You cannot change anything that you are not aware of. Therefore, education is the key. Educating yourself about what is normal or healthy for you is the only way to create awareness, and therefore, effective change. In her TED talk, Tasha Eurich discusses how there is a ton of research to show that the most self-aware people ask the question "what" significantly more than the question "why."[24] So "what can I do about it," is more productive and proactive than "why me?" This book aims to do that, to help you ask the right questions based on a more educated understanding of what is going on inside of you.

My message here is simple: understand what healthy means for you; find out what works for you and figure out how to make it happen. Find people who will help you make it happen. The empowered patient will bring this discussion, knowledge, and plan to their current medical professionals. Those you wish to treat you, will be the ones to agree and jump on board.

First, let's get a better understanding of what a "healthy you" looks like on you. Then, make a solid commitment to Change. Sounds easy, right? Well, if it was, the whole world would be healthy. I wouldn't be writing this book, nor would I have a job in healthcare.

Life is an adventure, a crazy, exciting, and often terrifying adventure. And what adventure is easy? As Theodore Roosevelt once said, *"Nothing in the world is worth having or worth doing unless it means effort, pain, difficulty… I have never in my life envied a human being who led an easy life. I have envied a great many people who led difficult lives and led them well.*"1 If a life well-lived is a struggle—as you know it is—then you might as well empower yourself to live it to the fullest. So, strap in and enjoy the ride! And know that you are never alone.

Is it Possible to Enjoy the Ride of Life?

I am honored and excited to begin this journey with you. I will be your guide on this adventure towards self-discovery and re-ownership of your healthcare. Throughout my twenty-plus years in healthcare, I have seen countless people rise, take back their health and reclaim their personal power through debilitating situations. It is possible to still have a vibrant, happy life despite chronic pain, brain injuries, cancer, car accidents, and surgeries. It takes motivation to change. It takes an empowered consumer of healthcare to navigate through the system.

We have learned to rely on healthcare professionals to care FOR us, rather than work WITH us. It is time we use the healthcare system for its intended purpose: to guide and educate us along this incredible journey called life. You need to be in the driver's seat and in charge of your decisions, actions, and choices. Your health care team advises; you act. Stop taking the back seat—a passive role—in your own healthcare. This is your reminder—and wakeup call—to action.

From my professional and personal experience, I know that the good majority of us are searching for this guidance on how to put selfcare back into the foundation of your health care. I have seen this approach work time and time again. Gaining a better understanding of how your body works and having a team to consult and guide you towards a solid selfcare plan works. This is the beginning, the catalyst, your invitation to get back in the driver's seat.

Take this journey with me. Explore what's holding you back. Learn how to surround yourself with strong, compassionate people. Build a team of healthcare professionals who will support you along your selfcare journey. Be empowered and enjoy every moment of this crazy ride we call life!

What Qualifies You to Be My Guide on this Journey?

"There are worse things to be than a disease," she said, idly thoughtful. "When you have one, it reminds you that you're alive. Makes you fight for what you have. When the disease has run its course, normal healthy life seems wonderful by comparison."
— *"The Way of Kings" pages 505-6*

I have a very unique perspective when it comes to health care and selfcare. First, I have worked as an occupational therapist in an outpatient clinic for over fifteen years. Most of those years have been spent working with a focus on what I call a whole body or whole health approach. The term "holistic" is now such a broad, overused term that it is often discounted in the healthcare world and thought of as non-credible. I chose to be an occupational therapist rather than a physical therapist due to the emphasis on treating the combined mental and physical health aspects of a person. The philosophy of occupational therapy addresses the person as a whole. It accepts that the mental and physical aspects of a person need to be addressed equally, for they affect each other. I have seen this in the clinical setting time and time again. A human without a purpose, an occupation or role, lacks hope and inner fire.

I am not a psychologist, or a doctor, and I do not pretend to be. This book is representative of the approach I have used, and seen work, over my past 20 plus years in my OT practice. The Matrix is an integration of all that I have learned from my interactions with other medical professionals, my patients, and my own personal experiences.

I own and operate a small outpatient rehab clinic, Motivate Therapy, where both occupational therapists and physical therapists alike treat the whole person. We approach each individual as such—as a whole individual, rather than a body part, a wrist patient, or a man with urinary incontinence. A shoulder dysfunction is never just about the shoulder. The shoulder is not separate from the head, neck, chest, or trunk. We look at—and treat—the whole picture with the end goal of guiding the person back towards their ultimate goal, which is to heal and improve their quality of life. Quality of life means different things to different people. Thanks to our unique approach and perspective, the clinic has gained a reputation for its ability to treat many different, complex problems.

My passion over the past fifteen years has led me to also become certified in Integrative Yoga Therapy, massage therapy, and pelvic floor therapy. So, most of my patients deal with chronic pain and pelvic floor issues. By pelvic floor, I refer to anything related to bowel, bladder, or sexual function. When these three functions are out of whack—believe me—your quality of life changes.

Too many people go through life thinking they must live with chronic pain, urinary incontinence, or low back pain. No doubt, you know someone who lives with one of those issues. And too often, doctors have told their patients that pain or dysfunction is either common or there is nothing they can do about it. People are told to learn to live with it, but they are never shown how.

Sex with a loved one should never be painful, and leaking urine or stool should never be okay. Despite what the commercials say, pee should never "just happen" without your control. Nor should knee pain with climbing stairs or gardening. You need to seek help, learn more, and then try everything there is to heal. No one should have to settle for a life not well-lived or even half-lived. You must seek to learn and try everything else first, before acceptance.

Why is Selfcare So Important to Healthcare?

I see our roles in healthcare—whether OT, PT, physicians, nurses, or any allied professional—as that of a guide. We study to learn how to best guide you toward your whole health potential. At least, we start out that way. But I see the healthcare profession shifting towards a place where people rely on us to fix them. As a patient, you are placed in the "protocol box," such as total knee rehab, or prolapse surgery. Once you plateau, the surgeon steps away or rehab ends, and you are on your own.

The medical profession needs to improve our role as your guides, but it begins with you. You need to help us help you find your way by taking back the reigns. By getting back into the driver's seat you will show your healthcare team that you are motivated to take back your health and live the life that you love. My conversation with each patient begins with, "What are your goals?" "How can we help you achieve them?" And then, "What are you doing to achieve them?" You are the leader and the goal setter.

Is it Possible to Live with Chronic Illness Using the Selfcare Matrix?

My unique perspective became even more unique when I was diagnosed with acute disseminate central nervous system Lyme disease two years ago. The "acute disseminate" part means that I had meningitis—or swelling in the brain and spinal cord—for at least four weeks before it was caught and treated. I have yet to completely recover and I still treat the symptoms. Even as I write this book I have had to stop and start again several times dealing with illness. Whether from the bacteria, or the side-effects of the medications, I am still fighting; fighting to accept what I can't change and fighting to change what I can. It is not a well-understood disease, so it has clarified my need to be my own healthcare advocate.

I am now on both sides of the trenches. I am a chronic illness patient and a therapist who specializes in chronic health issues. I have spent years teaching people the importance of finding a team of medical professionals that supports them through the healing process. And now I am fighting every day to find that same support.

After six months of fighting, I began to build a healthcare team that would support my beliefs; that would give me the guidance and resources that I needed to get my life back. Due to the nature of my job I am very fortunate to have had a small team of doctors that knew me prior to the disease and have supported me every step of the way. I found a Lyme-literate doctor, LLMD, who gave me more antibiotics, supplements, and resources which improved my health and gave me my life back. I believed in myself enough to listen to my gut and not take "it's in your head" for an answer.

My healthcare team includes a primary care physician (PCP), a Lyme-literate physician and/or a functional medicine doctor, an OT, PT, a psychologist, a gynecologist, and a dentist. I consult with an integrative primary care physician, and massage therapists. Friends and family complete the circle. All these support systems build me up when I'm down and share in my joy when I am up.

So, I fight; I fight every day. I fight to not give up; I fight to find the best team of people who will not give up on me either. I know at the end of the day—whether healthy or ill—I am doing the best that I can to care for myself. Yes, I have good days, great days, terrible days, and in-between days. And yes, there are days when I want to give up, too tired to fight. But I am alive, surrounded by people who love and support me, and I have a job that I love; a solid purpose on this earth. So, I am blessed many times over.

Do I wish that I had never contracted this disease? Heck, yeah! But I have made many delicious flavors of lemonade out of the "Lyme lemon."

I would not have written this book had I not been knocked on my butt and forced to look at my life and priorities. It gave me a different patient perspective and I believe it helped me become a better therapist. I also manage my business in a completely different, more efficient way. I have a lot of time to read and learn—time I never would have had if I hadn't been forced to stop working 50-60-hour weeks. So, yes, disease can be a blessing in disguise. It's all a matter of perspective.

PUT SELFCARE BACK INTO HEALTHCARE

"Self-care is never a selfish act—it is simply good stewardship of the only gift I have, the gift I was put on earth to offer others. Anytime we can listen to true self and give the care it requires, we do it not only for ourselves, but for the many others whose lives we touch."
— *Parker J. Palmer*

Now is the time to stopping thinking of your healthcare as a passive system of "they fix me" instead of "I fix or maintain myself." Your health is your responsibility and you have the power to heal. You have rights and responsibilities that you need to put back into your list of top priorities. Committing to daily selfcare as your top priority is your first step towards healing and feeling like a whole, vibrant person again.

"How do I do that?" you ask. Before we get into the specific steps, let's first define health. Let's also discuss the difference between healing and curing. Then we'll define, or re-define, what "selfcare" is and what it is not.

What is the Difference between Health, Healing and Curing?

Every person reading this will be in a different state of health. People rarely go to their doctor or come to physical or occupational therapy because they are feeling terrific. The same holds true for reading a book about how to heal yourself. I'm sure you would agree that beginning healthy habits before you become sick or injured is your best bet. But there is always hope, no matter what the state of your current health. The World Health Organization defines health in three ways:

i. *Health is an absence of impairment or disease.*

ii. *Health is more of a state that allows you to successfully cope with all the demands of daily life, while still implying the absence of disease or impairment.*

iii. *Health as a state of balance that you have established within yourself as well as within your physical and social environments.*[2]

The first definition talks about health as a lack of disease or impairment. So, you get sick, you go to the doctor, and say, "fix me." The second begins to imply that you play a role in your own health, but not until you are sick. The third definition discusses health as a *"state of balance between yourself and your environment."* For the purposes of this book, your "environment" will refer to your entire or whole body (biological, physical, mental, emotional, and spiritual), as well as within your world and community. The third definition of health is achievable by anyone, but only when done in balance with yourself and others.

Building your selfcare matrix means relying on yourself first and then a trusted team of people. You get to determine the members of that team. Whether you are terminally ill, have chronic pain, or are just trying to prevent disease or illness, it is possible to live a healthy, balanced life.

"Health is a state of balance that you have established within yourself as well as within your physical and social environments."

Now that we have established what health is, let's clarify healing. I used to think of healing and curing as the same thing and that I can't be "healed" unless I am "cured." One frustration I have experienced as an OT is working with a patient for six weeks and seeing them grow and change dramatically. But when I re-assess their progress and ask them how they are doing, they reply, "I'm not any better."

However, based on my objective testing, they have met 75% of their goals. They can walk and sit longer, play with their kids, and they no longer avoid grocery shopping. Their quality of life is improving, hooray! Yet, to them, they are "no better" because they still have pain or are "not like they were before." This is the frustration of healing.

If you are constantly comparing yourself to "how you were" versus "how you are now," you will always find fault. Change is the only constant in this life. If your only goal is to return to perfect health or how you were a year ago—which ultimately means not changing— you are setting yourself up for failure. Staying on this path will eventually lead to losing hope. Giving up on your own health potential is the same as spending months on a 10,000-piece puzzle where you misplace the last piece and decide to scrap the whole thing because it's too hard. Why waste your time looking for that last piece? Would you end a 20-year marriage because "it is not what it used to be," rather than working harder to make it better? To discover what is healthy and not healthy—now, today—that should be your goal. It will never be what it used to be, because life is about change and growth. You are worth the effort! Don't stop looking for answers; hold onto hope.

Healing ultimately means "becoming whole." This is not the same as "curing," which means to eliminate all evidence of disease.[3]

Talk to anyone who has had cancer and is now in remission or has been told that all evidence of the cancer is gone. They are "cured" of cancer, but they will tell you that their bodies are not the same. They may feel fantastic, function normally, and feel perfectly happy and content, but some things have changed. They may become tired more easily. Their skin may feel different, or their muscles may feel weaker. They may not be the same, but if they are content with their lives and feel that they have a good quality of life, then they are whole.

How Does Healing Mean Becoming Whole for Me?

Feeling whole or complete is a much more realistic goal. Expecting to be "cured" of any sign that the disease was there in the first place can set you up for failure. To feel whole again is to feel complete—physically, mentally, emotionally and spiritually. When we combine the definitions of healthy and healing, we become whole again (living in a state of balance within our bodies and interactions with others).

This is not a static process. This is something you should strive for daily. Every day you will wake up in a different state of health. This day is here for you to practice—again and again—how to find a balanced state of health; how to heal yourself. Perfection is not the goal, so let's take that word right out of your vocabulary. Daily awareness of how you feel and what you can do about it— that is your goal from moment to moment.

Know that you are never alone in this process.

Why Should We Re-Define Self-Care?

Self-care, much like the term 'health'—can have many different definitions. Let's explore three definitions from three different sources:

1. *Dictionary.com defines self-care as "...care of the self without medical or other professional consultation".*
   (http://www.dictionary.com/browse/self-care)[4]

2. *Wikipedia defines it as "Self-care... In health care, self-care is any necessary human regulatory function which is under individual control, deliberate and self-initiated. Some place self-care on a continuum with health care providers at the opposite end to self-care. In modern medicine, preventive medicine aligns most closely with self-care."*[5]

3. *Oxford dictionary states that it is "... The practice of taking action to preserve or improve one's own health. The practice of taking an active role in protecting one's own well-being and happiness, in particular during periods of stress."*[6]

All sources refer to self-care as a noun. I propose we use it as a verb, an action, a way to take an active role in your health and wellness. The first definition implies that self-care is to be independent of the healthcare system. The second refers to it as necessary to human function. The third definition refers to "taking action"—protecting your health and well-being, but only during periods of stress.

So, is self-care separate from healthcare? Is it a method to prevent the need for healthcare, or only necessary in case of an emergency? If self-care can be all these things, why can't we re-write and re-define it as "selfcare"; a verb defined as actively caring for one's self in all situations, every moment, every day, as an integrated part of healthcare; to listen to and act upon one's daily, whole health needs. Selfcare means to be a proactive, responsible team-member of your own health care; to use your resources and make the right choices for you.

Selfcare Redefined:

"Selfcare;" /verb/self.care/

1. *Actively caring for one's self in all situations, every moment, every day, as an integrated part of healthcare.*
2. *Listen to and act upon one's daily, whole health needs.*
3. *Be a proactive, responsible team-member of your own health care; use your resources, make the right choices for you and act accordingly.*

What is the Difference between Alternative and Integrative Health and Why Should it Matter to Me?

Let's now throw the term "alternative healthcare" right out the window. 'Alternative' suggests that you should choose either alternative medicine or western or allopathic medicine. Allopathic medicine is what we think of as standard healthcare; doctors, surgeons, PT and OT.[46] Complimentary alternative medicine, CAM, includes chiropractors, acupuncturists, and massage therapists. And yes, not everything is created equal. Every person will practice medicine differently. CAM services, as well as allopathic services, should be based on solid evidence that it works. Doing your research first is always necessary to ensure you are taking the right avenue for yourself. These services can and should work together, complement each other. They all need to be considered as part of an integrated plan to be effective.[47, 48]

Let's re-define medicine as an integrated approach between the patient and his or her team of professionals, rather than "western or allopathic medicine" versus "alternative or holistic medicine." You— the patient—and your team of professionals have the option to choose. Together, through intelligent, educated awareness, you decide which health approaches make sense. Then you begin healing your systems as a whole rather than as many different, separate parts.

What is Self-Healthcare and How Can it Help Me?

From here on out we will refer to this team approach as "self-health care." It is an integral concept within the Selfcare Matrix. With self-healthcare you cannot have one without the other. If you do not care for yourself, then you do not care for health. There is no "self" without "health." If your health fails, you die.

There is one thing and one thing only that we "own" in this life, and that is your body. And really, you are renting it, but it is yours and yours alone. It is the one and only true thing that you are in charge of until the very end. There is also no "I" in selfcare either. Self-healthcare relies on you as the driver. Yet, it is dependent on team support to be a successful working model. This insures the matrix adapts to your ever-changing health and wellness needs.

What Do I Not Have Permission to Do Within My Selfcare Matrix and Why?

As your self-appointed guide, I find that it's best to establish up front what self-healthcare is and what it is not. Clarifying the boundaries allows you to more clearly see the bigger picture. Then we can get on with the fun stuff; learning how to take back control of your healthcare.

Selfcare is NOT permission to:

1. **Doctor bash**. Every medical professional can have value along your healthcare journey. They each have very specific areas of expertise. They have dedicated their lives to learning their craft so that they may help the lives of others. They deserve respect. Even the medical professionals that do not guide you towards your goals, still teach you invaluable lessons. This helps you narrow down the types of practitioners that do not fit your needs, and the procedures or treatments you wish to avoid.

2. **Self-prescribe, self-diagnose, or self-treat** without good use of resources and educated advice.

3. **Rely on "Dr. Google."** Nothing will replace the power of human-to-human interaction for educated guidance and advice.

4. **Give up**. That would be the opposite of taking an active role in your health. Never say never. Keep on fighting, learning, and teaching yourself and others.

5. **Be a demanding, aggressive patient**. The human system is so complicated and no one—including you—can know everything. Being empowered means having an open-mind

and being open to the opinions and advice of others.

6. **Give up on the healthcare system.** Caring for yourself does not mean being completely alone on your journey or waiting until your health is in a dire state before seeking help.

7. **Blame or find fault in the actions of others.** We are not responsible for the actions of others, yet we are responsible for how we respond. Taking action, making good choices, and staying positive along your journey will set you up for success. Blaming others, including yourself, will only negatively affect all aspects of your health and goal success.

8. **Assume everything you read and hear is always true, applies to you and will work for you.** Everybody is different. Your body is unlike any other on earth as far as how it reacts to various health techniques (medications, surgery, therapy, exercise, food, etc.). Research can be a tricky thing to understand too.

What Are My Rights and Responsibilities?

Self-health care comes with rights and responsibilities. Below, you will find a general list that we hand out to every one of our patients when we first begin their therapy program. It relates to all self-healthcare.

- I am accountable for my choices and actions. I am responsible for the mistakes I make.
- I accept where I am today knowing it will change tomorrow.
- I accept and am committed to being myself.
- I will stop and take time for selfcare without feeling selfish. It is my health, my life, after all.

- I have the right to refuse requests without feeling selfish.
- I am responsible for communicating my needs; no one knows my body as well as I do.
- I am responsible for learning more.
- I have the option to choose my treatment and take responsibility for my choices.
- I am responsible for being, thinking and acting positively, realizing that when I practice being positive, I will become better at it. If I expect catastrophe, that's what I'll get.
- I have the right to be confident in myself and in those around me.
- I am an empowered consumer of my own healthcare.
- I am responsible for understanding my health insurance benefits.
- I have the right to be competent and proud of my accomplishments.
- I have the right to feel and express frustration and ask for help with problem-solving.
- I have the right to be treated as a capable adult.
- I have the right to be safe, feel respected, and receive dignified care always.
- I have the right and responsibility to find a team of like-minded health care professionals that I know, like, and trust.
- I must listen, respect, and trust my chosen healthcare team.
- I am responsible for using my resources wisely and sharing what I learn with others.
- I am responsible for trying new things responsibly and discussing my findings with my team.

- I have the right and responsibility to ask questions.
- I am responsible for taking an active role in my healing.
- I have the right to choose how I live and how I die; hope and happiness are a choice.
- I understand that healthcare does not end after my health team appointment.
- My needs are as important as the needs of others.
- I have the right to grow, learn, change, and value my age and experience.
- I have the right to change my mind.
- I have the right to say, "I don't know," but am responsible for being open to learning more.
- I have the right to disagree.
- I have the right to say, "I don't understand."
- I have the right to say, "I hurt."
- I have the right to say, "I am worried it will hurt me."
- I am responsible for "actively" attending and participating in my healthcare sessions.
- I am responsible for "actively" participating in my home program, (including taking my medications or doing my home exercise program).
- I am responsible for being truthful, open, and honest with daily follow-through of my therapist's and physician's recommendations.
- I am responsible for recognizing and respecting the rights of other patients and staff.
- I am responsible for promoting my own safety by becoming an active, involved, and informed member of my healthcare team.

What Does Committing to Selfcare Mean for Me and How Can it Change My Life?

Once you have committed to making selfcare a daily choice, you will see your healthcare team in a new light. All members of your healthcare team are experts in their fields, but how you use them is up to you. They will guide and advise you, but you get to make the ultimate decision.

As an OT guiding patients toward whole body health, I have heard many times, "Why didn't my doctor send me here years ago?"

If you are given advice that doesn't work for you, then it is up to you to keep searching. You get to choose which therapy clinic to attend based on what is best for you. That is why surrounding yourself with people you know, like, and trust is so important. And then using them, ask questions and do your research.

Your team should recommend what is best for you, based on your goals, medical findings and past medical history—not what is financially best for them or their institution. And "googling" something can help you learn more but using resources such as people who have dealt with and are successfully living with similar symptoms is going to give you a more realistic and successful outcome. Sharing what has worked for you, giving positive reviews to healthcare professionals online or in surveys, is so incredibly important. We are all on this journey together. So, what is stopping you from healing and living a vibrant life?

TRY THIS: Selfcare and Me

- *Name three ways you do "selfcare" every day. Selfcare is something just for you. For me, it means going for a walk or spending ten minutes a day just talking with my husband about nothing; it's also writing in my journal, taking 30-second "breathing breaks" (everyday). No self-criticism if you can't think of anything or if you do less than that. Stick to it, you will have a long list eventually.*

- *Write down three daily selfcare ideas on a piece of paper and place them somewhere where you will see them daily. Commit to practicing these ideas every day. Some of the things that I do include:*
  - *Smiling to myself when I wake up*
  - *Reaching out a friend*
  - *Stretching five minutes a day*
  - *Walking 30 minutes a week*
  - *Reading a positive affirmation or quote every night.*

Circle one and commit to doing that one thing every day. Place it somewhere where you will see it every day, such as on your bathroom mirror. Change it daily, weekly, or monthly.

PRINCIPLE #2:

IDENTIFY WHAT'S HOLDING YOU BACK

"Not until we are lost do we begin to understand ourselves."

— *Henry David Thoreau*

Why Does Mindset Matter?

Before creating and committing to new habits, it is important to establish up front what your mindset is when it comes to learning and growing. In Carol Dwecks' book, "Mindset: The New Psychology of Success," she discusses that there are two ways of thinking about our intelligence and possibility for growth. There is the "fixed mindset" or the "growth mindset." I know that I used to think that a person's IQ is what defined their intelligence; whether they were smart or not. That the IQ test was the end-all and be-all of measuring intelligence. We are born with a certain amount of intelligence, from our genes or upbringing, and that's it. That is considered a "fixed mindset." A mental statement of a person with a fixed mindset would be "I can't do it." However, a person with a growth mindset sees a challenge or failure as a learning opportunity. This mindset takes the statement "I can't do it" and turns it into "I can't do it, **yet**."[26, 27]

Decide now which mindset you will choose going forward. It will make all the difference in your successful outcome of achieving your selfcare goals, creating new habits and finding the right healthcare team for you.

Choose not to get stuck in the mire of self-limiting
beliefs. You have limitless potential. Always.

How Are Reasons Different from Excuses?

Let's establish right from the start that this is a judgment-free zone. I am a patient and a healthcare team member, so I have both used and heard plenty of excuses. I have done it and will do it again soon. But knowing, admitting, and not accepting it all the time is where your power lies. We need to call ourselves out. We need to hold up the mirror and examine both our healthy and not-so healthy habits. Not to judge and abuse ourselves, but to learn and grow. How else are we ever going to change and make better decisions? Admitting the need to change is what will empower you to act.

So, what's the difference between an excuse and a reason? Pure and simple, it's accountability.

An excuse is an explanation for why something is the way it is that always involves the blame being put on a situation or someone else. You have the knowledge, ability, and understanding about how and why you need to make the right choice. Yet, instead of doing the right thing, you choose otherwise, and blame others for your choices and the consequences. That, my friend, is an excuse.

A reason is an explanation for why something is the way it is with everyone involved taking accountability or responsibility for his or her part in a situation. If you fail to do something due to circumstances that are completely out of your control, then you have a reason.[8]

Have You Used Them?

"When you are upset, remind yourself the cause of your discomfort is your own attitude. This is freedom."

— *Unknown*

Most people who are familiar with it know that Lyme disease is not a well-understood disease. There is so much controversy about the bacteria and treatment options. There is a huge disconnect between practitioners and too often, the patients suffer. The Center for Disease Control has a specific protocol for "acute" Lyme disease. Their common stance is that it is cured within thirty days of medical treatment, according to a Lyme-expert physician with whom I spoke. Any lasting symptoms or diagnosis of Lyme after thirty days is considered chronic. Yet, according to the CDC, there is no such thing as "chronic Lyme disease."

I was diagnosed "acute disseminate Lyme disease" two to four weeks after the initial infection. Yet, as of now, I have been dealing with symptoms for almost two years. I have lots of excuses and reasons to blame the CDC and the medical community for the fact that my life has been turned upside down. I no longer have the exact same quality of life that I did two years ago. My reason for my current health situation is that no one healthcare practitioner understands this disease. Lyme disease presents itself differently in every person. There are many reasons for the disconnect within the medical community about Lyme and other chronic illnesses, but there are many professionals looking at those reasons and researching better solutions. They may be the minority but there are people within the medical community trying to make everyone within the system more accountable for delivering workable solutions and better diagnostic testing.

However, if I were to let my health and healing end here, then I would be using excuses. And believe me I could give you a ton of excuses and blame a lot of people and entities for my many bad days. But where would that get me?

Have You Heard Them?

On the other side of the coin, as a therapist, I think that I have heard just about every excuse out there is as to why selfcare is impossible or inconvenient. Why selfcare won't change anything. And yes, some have good reasons when the medical community is unable to diagnose or explain why things are the way they are. But selfcare does not end with reasons; it ends with excuses. An excuse is just that—a disguised reason to not be responsible for acting and to give up. When it is someone or something else's fault, then you have permission to ignore the problem.

"Selfcare does not end with reasons; it ends with excuses."

No, selfcare does not end with a reason—that is where it begins. Once you get answers—such as "it's cancer," or "we don't know what it is, so you need to learn how to live or cope with it"—your action plan for selfcare begins. Ultimately, PT and OT should be about holding up the mirror, helping people become more aware as to what current habits are contributing to their health, and which habits are not. Then we need to teach them what to change, and how to maintain that awareness for a lifetime.

First, you must understand what habits and thinking patterns are not healthy and are holding you back. Tim Ferris coined the term "fear-setting" instead of goal-setting. He suggests first separating what you can control from what you can't control. This can decrease emotional reactivity and allows you to be more proactive and positively affect change in yourself.[9]

Once you can see the chains blocking you from growth, you'll also be able to see the key that unlocks them. Then it's all about commitment. Ha! Easier said than done, right? Hmmm... another excuse?

Do You Use Every Excuse in the Book?

Let's explore some of the many excuses, (or self-limiting beliefs) that you may have used—or are currently using—as well as different ways to look at them. You are setting yourself up for failure by giving your excuses power. Accepting excuses and having a fixed mindset is like being stuck in the mud.

As I mentioned earlier, Tasha Erich's research has shown that people who are successfully self-aware, use the question "what" more often than "why." She also found that constant "introspection," or examining your own thoughts and feelings, can lead to depression. So, examine your excuses with a positive and open-mind. Are they limiting your health potential? Change your statements and put a more constructive and proactive spin on them. This will help unstuck you from the mud in order to take forward steps.

Excuses are statements easily ignored. Acknowledging that you are using excuses is the first step. You can easily walk away from an excuse. But turn that excuse into a question, answer it, and you have a goal waiting to be conquered. Ignoring the problem and being passive is no longer an option once you have an answer. Try exchanging "why" questions with "what" whenever possible. This will eventually lead to goal-setting. I have given you lots examples below.

Excuse: "I don't have the time."

Suggested Questions:

- *What am I choosing to spend my time on and does it lead to my health and happiness?*
- *What can I do to make the time?*
- *How much time do I actually need?*
- *What is stopping me from taking the time to take care of my own needs?*
- *Do I have the time to take care of other people's needs?*
- *Can anyone help me? If so, why haven't I asked?*
- *What are my expectations?*

I started with the "no time" excuse for a reason. It is the most common excuse out there, because we all use it instead of acknowledging that we either don't know where to start or how to do what we need to do. Too often we just do not make ourselves a priority. If you truly believe that you do not have the time to be and stay healthy, consider how you are prioritizing your time. How much is "enough" time to dedicate to your health and well-being?

To be blunt, you must make time. You are making time to read this book. Bingo! Selfcare in action! Look at you go!

Start getting up earlier. Lie on the floor and stretch while watching TV in the evening with your family. Try taking a few slow conscious breaths in the car at the stoplight. Drink water before you reach for junk food. Jump rope with your kids while they are playing outside.

There is time. You must make it a priority and you must make yourself accountable.

That's the joy of therapy. We give the patient a home program. They come back and feel bad that they didn't do it, even though they knew we were going to ask. Feeling badly catches up with you eventually and it can be very motivating.

After two to three weeks of feeling guilty, the patient either gives up— "I don't have the time to do my exercises, so therapy is not worth it"— or they give it a try, and consistently do their exercises as prescribed for two weeks in a row. They are amazed at how much better they feel. Viola! That excuse becomes a reason for selfcare.

REALITY CHECK: You must be realistic. Single parenting without support, working third shifts, running your own business, and life in general does make it more difficult to find time. But 10-15 minutes still counts as time spent on selfcare. And use your resources. People do want to help.

Excuse: "I don't have the money."

Suggested Questions:

- *How can I rearrange my financial priorities and make selfcare my first priority?*
- *Are there other cheaper or better solutions out there that are more flexible?*
- *Can I talk to them (gym, clinic) about a payment plan?*

- *What am I currently choosing to spend my money on that is not as important as my health and healing?*

True story. I worked with a patient who suffered for years with—what she thought was—chronic urinary tract infections. She constantly felt the urge to pee. You know how it feels when you are stuck on the highway and need to pee so badly but there is no exit for another 60 minutes? Well, imagine feeling that even after you go to the bathroom. Now, imagine living your life like that all day every day.

And when you think it's your organ—your bladder, kidney or urethra—you think that you can't do anything about it. Once your doctor says that the test shows all those organs are healthy, one tends to give up. After several years of going from doctor to doctor, she found one that recommended pelvic floor therapy.

She came to my clinic. She had a $7,000 deductible. She had just moved. Her kids were in several sports, so money was tight. She decided to come one time every two to four weeks and pay out of pocket. Once she started feeling better, she realized that her health should be the priority. She found a team of health care professionals that cared, listened, and guided her towards wellness.

She found ways to feel better. She cut down on the kids' activities. She made some changes in her budget. She found a way to come once a week so that she could get better faster and learn how to manage her symptoms and live the life that she wanted to live. She learned drinking water and managing her stress completely changed her life. That's money and time well spent.

Excuse: "My insurance will only allow me to..."
(see this doctor / go to this clinic / only take a
medication other than the prescribed medication).

Suggested Questions:

- *What can I do to get what I need? Have I talked to my insurance company?*
- *Have I talked to at least two to three different reps at my insurance company?*
- *Have I tried an appeal process?*
- *Have I tried a different medication in the same prescribed class, after discussing it with my physician?*
- *Have I asked my doctor or clinic of choice about payment plans?*
- *What are my other options?*

Don't ever take the first answer from your insurance company as written in stone. Understanding your insurance benefits is your responsibility. But the advice you receive can be interpreted in different ways by different people. And appeal processes do work, take it from me.

Many healthcare providers verify your healthcare benefits as a courtesy. They call and talk to someone to find out if they are in network with your plan, and what it covers for a certain procedure or therapy. But they don't always get the whole story. You should always call and check for yourself. The answers can and do often vary based on whom you talk to and how much information you have to give. Even if you are not "in-network" and must pay out of pocket, do not let it end there. This is where your rights and responsibilities continue.

True Story: To get the answers I needed, I had to go to a "Lyme-literate" clinic. I had to pay out of pocket for everything. Labs, doctor appointments, and even the recommended medications were out-of-pocket expenses. So, I paid what I could, set up a plan for the rest, and sent every receipt that I had to the insurance company. And before taking the clinic's word for it, I called my insurance and asked them, "Do I have to pay out of pocket for this medication and procedure?" They guided me on how to do it in a way that would be covered at 100%. Had I not acted, I would never have known.

Excuse: "I'm too sick" or "My current state of health doesn't allow me to..."

Suggested Questions:

- *What am I able to do independently? How can I do more of it?*
- *What makes me happy?*
- *What am I currently able to do that I am not taking advantage of?*
- *Do I have support?*
- *Can I ask for help?*
- *How can I keep fighting in a way that does not stop me from doing the things that I love?*

It is so easy to overlook what we can do right now. Too often we can get stuck in "catastrophic thinking," choosing to focus on what we can't do. In nursing homes, OT's work with patients to dress, toilet, brush their hair and teeth in the morning. Simple things, like dressing, most of us do without thinking about it. However, for these patients it could take them an hour of painstaking effort to simply get dressed.

But they fight to do it independently every day because that is what they have left. And they are thankful for those abilities.

It is so important to appreciate what we do have, what we can do. Even if you are terminally ill, or maybe especially if you are terminal, selfcare is still essential. You deserve to be happy and to feel honored and heard. Revel in what you can do and ask for help when needed. There are so many emotions and physical changes going on that you need daily support. Whether this is from your friends and family or your medical support system, if you don't ask, they won't tell.

Be proactive in your how you live and how you die. If you are bedridden, what do you enjoy? Being surrounded by family? Having books read to you? Hearing nature? This warrants a discussion with your loved ones now while you're healthy. What would you want if you were on your deathbed and couldn't communicate? Discuss what makes you happy in realistic ways. "I'm too sick" is often used as an excuse for non-terminal patients as well.

Excuse: "I'm in too much pain. It will only make me worse,"
or "I have no hope" or "I have tried everything."

Suggested Questions:

- *What is your worst fear about this?*
- *What is the worst that can happen?*
- *How do I know if I never try?*
- *Have I asked others in my circle of trust what has helped them?*
- *What makes me happy?*
- *What am I good at?*
- *What would I like to get better at?*

- *Where does my "hope" come from?*
- *Is there anyone in my life that I admire and has a positive attitude?*

The same questions apply here as to the previous question. As we will soon discuss, understanding how your biological, mental, emotional, spiritual, and physical bodies are connected is so essential to your selfcare success. You will see how negative or "catastrophic" thinking will only land you in more negative situations, and more illness. Yes, you might have more pain, but if you do not try, you will still be in pain.

The more you take back control of your self-health care, the more confident you will become, because you are in control of every moment. That is choice. Moving and doing, being active in life, will always bring more joy than sitting around the house and isolating yourself from the world.

Keep fighting to live. Be around loving, positive people. Get involved. Do what you love or explore until you find out what you do love. Speak out, read or write a book, sit in the sun, volunteer, give back.

Excuse: "It's not my fault."

Suggested Questions:

- *So, what am I going to choose to do about it?*
- *Is it a legitimate excuse to give up?*
- *What can I learn from this? How can I apply this lesson to the rest of my life?*
- *What attitude am I choosing?*
- *What are my choices?*

Yes, you may have been in a bad car accident or surgical accident and that's horrible. Yes, it was someone else's fault. But now you get to choose what to do about it. Blaming others only sucks the life out of you; it does not contribute to your health. It only gives you an excuse to stay in the same place. And yes, that may be comfortable and familiar, but there will be no growth. If you practice hate and blame, you will excel at it. Practice forgiveness and responsibility and you will heal and become a beacon of light for others.

Example: I am so inspired by the "Wounded Warriors." These men and women chose to go into harmful situations to protect our freedom. They return home as completely changed individuals. They are in wheelchairs, missing limbs, and/or suffer post-traumatic stress syndrome. But if you've ever seen them speak, you'll see that they strive to accept it and keep on fighting. They see it as another challenge to conquer; a new mission in life. Never give up. Accept your choices, appreciate life and keep fighting. That is their message.

Example: In society, urinary incontinence has been an accepted symptom after giving birth to children. Yet, I see patients every day that do not accept it, although their doctors told them to do their Kegels or that leaking is normal. They do their research and find other options, such as pelvic floor therapy. Same thing with women who have pain with intercourse. They are often told that it is normal for sex to hurt. They do not accept it, so they stay proactive. They research or talk to their friends. They take back control so that they can go shopping with confidence or be intimate with their spouse (and enjoy it). They determine what they want to live with and what they don't.

Excuse: "It will never work, and/or my doctor/
friend/colleague said it will never work."

Suggested Questions:

- *How do I know that for a fact?*
- *Am I willing to give up on myself before I even try?*
- *What do I have to lose by trying?*
- *Have I talked to several other trusted sources that have tried it and have failed?*

Everybody reacts differently so there is never a sure-fire way to know that whatever it is, won't work for you until you try.

Example: I once had a patient who said that she couldn't stand to be touched because the skin on her upper body was so sensitive. She described her pain as 10/10 all the time. She refused to try manual or massage therapy due to fear of pain with touch. She consulted with a therapist at my clinic first, and after three sessions, her pain was gone. She was learning the why and how about her condition, and now has hope for the first time in ten years. She had been told by several members of her medical team that it was "in her head." You'll never know until you try.

Excuse: "I've tried everything else."

Suggested Questions:

- *Am I 100% sure that I have tried everything that has worked for my symptoms in all other cases?*
- *Have I talked to trusted sources about what they have tried and where they have gone?*

- *Have I addressed healing all the systems of my body (biological, physical, emotional, mental, social and spiritual health)?*
- *Do I have a strong healthcare team that I know, trust and like? If not, what can I do about it?*

Remember that everyone is fighting his or her own battles. Even those that seem happy and healthy have worked with medical team members in the past. Ask them what helped. Read reviews. Look for the positive ones. No pill, surgery, doctor, therapist, clinic, rehab, hospital is created equal. Medical professionals are humans too and we all excel at different things. Do not let your selfcare journey end just because you have tried several different options and they have yet to work as you expected. You just must keep looking, talking, trying, and learning.

I treated a gentleman who had been experiencing pelvic pain for years. He had severe pain in the muscles that he sits on, as well as constant abdominal pain. As is the case with most of our patients with chronic pain, he had been to several doctors as well as PT/OT clinics, tried injections and drugs, and nothing was helping. He talked to medical professionals that he trusted as well as friends and family. He did not give up, and finally found a physician who referred him to pelvic floor therapy. We discussed what worked, what didn't work and explored treatment options that he had not yet tried. He reports that he is 90% better and enjoys life again, including his job that requires sitting all day.

Excuse: "It hurts when I do this."

Suggested Questions:

- *What can I do that doesn't hurt?*

- *Have I tried moving every body part, not just the painful body part? Have I tried different positions such as standing, sitting, lying down?*
- *Have I tried different environments such as walking in water versus on a solid surface or uneven surfaces?*
- *Does it still hurt if I am distracted or not thinking about the body part?*
- *Does the time of day matter? If I am stressed or fatigued?*

Finding what doesn't hurt and what feels good is the trick to re-training your mind and body. Don't give up. Finding a team that supports you, encourages you, and guides you towards self-discovery is your light at the end of tunnel. It is there. Don't let excuses blind you from seeing your own limitless potential.

Excuse: "I have kids, big family (that take up my time)…"

Suggested Questions:

- *What do I do with my limited alone time?*
- *What can I do to make more alone time?*
- *Do I have a spouse, partner, or supportive family member who can help me out 30 minutes a day or even every few days?*
- *Do my kids ever sleep, go to school or daycare?*
- *What happens to my kids when I am sick?*
- *What will happen to my kid if I become debilitated from lack of selfcare?*

Ah, yes, the kids excuse. The guilt card seems to be implanted with the egg once we become mothers and fathers. Suddenly, becoming a caregiver trumps all else. Yet, if you take a step back, you will see that being a healthy, happy parent makes for a happy, healthy family. Making yourself a priority not only helps you manage stress, but goal setting helps you manage your day. By taking care of yourself, you are also setting a good example for your children as they grow. Teaching them that selfcare is healthcare will begin the trend toward self-empowerment and accountability.

Excuse: "I don't like my doctor (or therapist, psychologist) and/or my doctor doesn't listen."

Suggested Questions:

- *Have I talked to my doctor about this openly and honestly?*
- *If I don't feel like I can talk to my doctor, have I tried speaking to the nurse who takes my blood pressure and checks me in?*
- *Have I tried asking other members of my doctor's team for the best ways to communicate with him or her or whether they know someone else who might be a good fit for me?*
- *What can I do to change the situation so that it best suits my healthcare needs?*

"Three strikes and you're out" can apply here. If you have been open and honest with your doctor and attempted communicating your needs and there is no change, you now have a reason to change team members. This is where reason versus excuses, setting boundaries, as well as positive attitude and realistic expectations come in. Both parties are accountable for their behaviors, actions, and choices. Communication is the key principle here.

Healthcare practitioners are expected to work on a very limited time schedule while taking notes in explicit detail so that your chart passes an insurance audit and to prevent mistakes. It does take skill to switch mental gears from the last patient to you. They are to remember that you are a person and not a patient; hear, listen, type, chart, and make the right decisions for you. And it is easier on some days. You do not know what is going on with that healthcare team member. He or she is also a human being. You don't know what happened in the room before you entered, or what their personal stress level is like on that day.

If you don't feel heard or you feel he or she has one foot out the door, they deserve to hear this from you so that they have the chance to change. If you discuss this with them more than two or three times, give them every opportunity to be more present, compassionate, and aware and nothing changes, then the accountability is on you. Find someone who will give you the presence and compassion that you deserve. If the normal way you drive to work is always an easy drive until one day a tree blocks the road, you must take a detour until you call to get it fixed. You don't stop taking that route. You go back once the road is fixed.

Excuse: "Surgery and pills helped in the past."

Suggested Questions:

- *What is stopping me from trying a natural or conservative method of healing?*
- *What aspect of the illness did the pills or surgery help and what did they not help?*
- *Why is the condition back?*
- *How did I feel taking pills? Did I experience side effects?*

- *Can I function normally on the pills?*
- *Do I remember what surgical recovery was like?*
- *How old was I when I last had surgery?*
- *What is my current state of health versus the last time?*

Your state of health going into surgery can define how you recover. Surgery and pills are often necessary, but it should not end there. Gone are the "fix me and forget it" days. You are still responsible for the health of your "container"—your physical body. Walking, exercising, stretching, and strengthening under the guidance of an expert in muscles, and nerves (i.e.; therapy such as PT/OT) will give you a better chance of recovering and maintaining the surgical outcomes. And the more you gain control of the habits that tip over your balanced health, the less you will have to rely on certain medications, such as painkillers and anti-inflammatory drugs.

Excuse: "I don't believe I can change."

Suggested Questions:

- *What is stopping me from trying?*
- *What specifically can't I change?*
- *What am I afraid of?*
- *Give examples as to how this has been true for me in the past.*
- *Am I the same person, with the same habits, state of health that I was one year, or 5-10 years ago?*
- *Do I enjoy practicing negativity? Has it worked well for me in the past?*
- *What is the worse that would happen if I tried saying "I believe I can change" everyday?*

Guess what? You've changed, whether you like it, know it or not. Change happens either way. Would you rather get to choose how you change and live your life in the face of inevitable change? This statement is the same as saying "I don't believe in myself." Growth does not come from negative thinking. Rearranging this statement to say, "I don't know how to change yet" is the beginning to learning how. If you don't know how to do something, yet you are motivated, then you begin learning. Talking to knowledgeable people is a great start. That is a "growth mindset." [26]

Excuse: "I don't have any motivation."

Suggested Questions:

- *What has motivated me in the past?*
- *What do I enjoy doing now?*
- *What happens when, (not if), injury or illness stops me from being able to do what I enjoy?*

This is all about the power of you. Motivation to survive is in your DNA. If you've lived this long, there is a reason. Looking at it from an evolutionary standpoint, your body is working how it should to survive and reproduce. From a spiritual standpoint, you still have something left to do on this earth. Being proactive vs. reactive means that you will care for your health now rather than when illness or injury takes you down. And believe me when I say, the former is WAY easier than the latter.

*Excuse: "I don't like (the taste of water, to exercise,
going to them gym / you fill in the blank)..."*

Suggested questions:

- *What type of movement do I like?*
- *What healthy habits do I currently have or had in the past that made me feel good?*
- *What brings me joy?*
- *Have I done anything consistently enough to truly know whether I like it or don't like it?*
- *Once I have been doing something consistently, how did it make me feel?*

Not liking something is not a REASON to not try it; it's an excuse. I have heard the "I don't like the taste of water" excuse my entire career. Yet, time and time again, once people constantly drink water, 90% of them learn to like it because they feel better when they drink it. Why? Because our bodies, biologically, need it to survive.

I am sure I missed many more excuses, but you get the point. Once you recognize an excuse for what it is, stand back and look at it. Change the question from a "why" to a "what" whenever possible. What is true and real? Is it truly a physical limitation or is the "ego" voice in my head telling me lies? Am I trying to get out of doing what I know is good for me? Is it my body or my mind doing the talking? What your mind wants and what your body needs can often differ. And they both can heal differently, on their own timelines.

You can have control of both, but only once you learn to hear and listen to what your body is telling you. Then you will have success at understanding how your thinking patterns can hold you back. Only then can you take charge and make positive changes. This is otherwise known as putting selfcare back into healthcare.

Try This: Turning Excuses into Questions

Write down every fear, reason, or excuse that you have used in the past about your selfcare goals. You can make columns for each selfcare topic, such as losing weight, being in an unhealthy relationship, or not exercising. Then go back and circle the ones that you do have control over—those are your excuses. Turn the excuses—or circled statements—into questions and answer them. You now have a place to start once you plan and set goals.

PRINCIPLE #3:

COMMIT TO CHANGE

"We delight in the beauty of the butterfly, but rarely admit the changes it has gone through to achieve that beauty."

— *Maya Angelou*

What Do You Value?

It bears repeating that you cannot change anything that you are not aware of. Admit it: change can be terrifying. Here, CHANGE represents the foundational principles of the Selfcare Matrix. It is the base from which you will build your daily selfcare goals, make decisions and measure your success. It is how you will determine the best new selfcare habits to make and who you want on your healthcare team.

CHANGE is the acronym for the principles, or core values, of the selfcare matrix. It is your personal guideline—or checklist—that will make daily selfcare choices simple and easy. But simple is never easy when first learning, so be patient with yourself. Perfection is never the goal; self-awareness is.

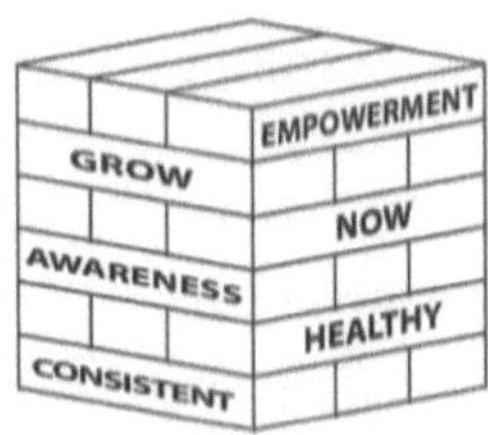

core values of CHANGE

CHANGE= Consistent. Healthy. Awareness. Now. Grow. Empowerment.

Applying these core values as the basis to your daily selfcare means that you are tapping into your whole-body potential every day. The CHANGE values will help create a path for you to follow and help guide you back when you stray. Let's break it down in a way that will allow you to make achievable, daily selfcare goals.

Think of any habit that you are currently doing (drinking coffee every morning, running three times a week, or only going to a walk-in clinic when you are very ill). And then answer these questions:

*Is it something that makes you **consistently** feel **healthy** based on self-**awareness** whenever you check in here and **now,** moment by moment? Will it help you **grow** forward? Does it leave you feeling grateful and **empowered**?*

Consistent: Is That Even Possible?

The definition of consistency is to constantly adhere to the same principle. It relates greatly to our habits, especially automatic reactions and how you act and react every day. One of my favorite sayings is that, "We are not meant to be perfect, we are meant to be whole," a quote by Jane Fonda. This is extremely important to remember when practicing consistency.

Your ego, that annoying voice in your head that fills you with self-doubt, will try to convince you that you are a failure, often even before you try. That is why we first looked at all the excuses that could possibly hold you back. The excuses and self-doubt are way easier to come by than positive affirmations from which achievable goals are born.

You will fail at being consistent. Nobody is perfect and that is not the goal. First, you must set an objective goal that you are sure to be successful at, such as "I will drink one glass of water every day before lunch." And every day, check it off your goal list. You will never know if something is a healthy habit for you until you do it—consistently—for at least a few weeks. If you stick with it and feel better—healthy habit, check. If you don't feel any better—lesson learned, nothing lost. Let failure inspire growth.

Ask yourself: Am I consistently making healthy choices today? What healthy habit category do I want to be more consistent with this month, physical or biological? Walk more or eat more vegetables?

Healthy: How Do I Consistently Make Healthy Choices Inside and Out?

Healthy outlook AND input. Just the word "healthy" often makes people cringe. We hold ourselves to such high standards that are impossible to reach. Now that you are committed to establishing consistent habits, let's assess whether they are healthy habits.

Remember that perfection is not the goal; being whole is. What you think and project on the outside is just as important as what you put inside of your mind and body.

I love the image of water flowing inside of a riverbed. Water flows over obstacles. It does not stop to say "Oh! There is a rock in my way! I don't have the energy to deal with this today or beat myself up for the way I approached the rocks yesterday or ten years ago." The river simply flows. When you drop a rock in a pond, ripples occur because you have changed the floor or foundation of the pond. So, how we think or speak to ourselves and how we portray ourselves to the world should take the same approach. You cannot always prepare for the rocks or curves ahead, but you can choose to approach it with a positive outlook. Approach your day with gratitude for life. Or tell yourself in the mirror that you are beautiful inside and out. That attitude will create positive ripples in your own life as well as improve the lives of others. And it is always one day—one moment—at a time.

Drinking water is the #1 best and easiest way to nourish our roots from the inside out. Now, if you are thinking that you hate the taste of water, I probably lost you at "easy." You are not just what you eat, but also what you drink. Water is the basis of all life, and that includes your body. The human adult body is comprised of about 60% water. The lungs that provide oxygen to your body are 83% water. Your brain—the control center of your entire body—is 73% water.[29] It is the most important nutrient needed by our body. You don't drink, you die. Research shows that "effects of water on daily performance and short and long-term health are quite clear," for all our bodily functions. There are few negative effects of water intake and the evidence of positive effects is quite clear from the literature."[28] The jury is still out about how much water a person should drink so do what feels best for you. Don't wait to feel thirsty; by the time you do, you are often already dehydrated.

Throughout my years as an OT, I have seen so many patients that have had constipation for most of their lives. Once they committed to healthy habits, primarily drinking more water, they will tell you their lives changed dramatically.

Healthy Habit 101: Drinking Water

Eating healthy is also an important topic to discuss here. The word "diet" is slowly being replaced with "healthy lifestyle." And there are so many lifestyle choices out there that it is easy to be confused and just say "forget it!" But again, consistency is key. Paying attention to what you put into your body will have a huge impact on how you feel, think, and act on a day-to-day basis. Pay attention to how you feel physically after eating fast food. Compare that to your energy levels and attitude after eating a healthier meal.

Balanced habits are healthy habits. Try to balance your day-to-day activities with exercise paired with stretching. Drink coffee, but also water. Eat healthy during the day, but also allow a treat in the afternoon. Clean the house, but also do meditation or breathing and relaxing exercises. Working because you have to with finding joy in what you do. Combining consistency with healthy habits and choices is the foundation for self-care. Now all you have to do to is to bring awareness to how your habits and choices affect the function of your whole body.

Question to ask yourself: What is the least healthy habit that I practiced yesterday? The healthiest? How did I feel after each one? How do I know it is a healthy habit? What aspect of my health do I know that I can improve today?

Awareness: Do I Really Have the Know-How?

This is the most important concept to practice every day if you ever want to get on and stay on the path towards health and wellness. This book really is about teaching you the "why" behind your body's signals so that you can understand how to change your current habits into healthy ones. Or you can create new ones. But to "know how" you need to "know why." Life is a tremendous book

First thing to understand is that your body is brilliant. From the beginning of life, your body is wired to preserve itself. It will protect itself at all costs. It is designed to always work in balance, in a state homeostasis.

How you walk, stand, and move by the time you are forty is an accumulation of the slips, falls, surgeries, sleep positions, work movements, sports and car accidents that you have had up to that point. So, it's probable that when you stand you clench at least one body part such as your left butt cheek, and your right shoulder. And you are most likely completely unaware of it.

Two things I hear many of my patients say, no matter their diagnosis, is "I do not know how to relax" and "I am not very flexible." Whether we look at these statements literally or figuratively, they are HUGE statements. And ultimately, obstacles towards taking control of our own health. To remove the obstacles, take these statements and turn them into "what" statements. This will begin to improve your self-awareness skills. "What can I do to become more flexible? What part of my life can I make more flexible? What situations do I find most relaxing?"

You are aware that relaxing and being flexible are difficult, but why don't you DO anything about it? It is often because you don't know how to change or where in your day to make time for it. You think that you must make specific times to relax or be more flexible. Yes, eventually this would be a great goal. But the easiest thing to change, and really the only time that matters, is right now. If you work on it right now, how can you fail?

Sitting here reading this, notice what your shoulders are doing. Are they elevated toward your ears? How about jaw tension? Check in with your buttocks muscles. How about your toes? Chances are—just by reading this and checking in with your body—some physical part of you relaxed. Something let go. Being aware of the here and now and the effects that it has on your body is the best way to create changes that matter. Creating a new norm or a new habit happens one moment at a time. That's it. You did it. You were aware by simply being present.

Habits that create non-healthy movement patterns often happen for the right reason. Our bodies are protecting us from possible repetitive injury or helping to heal from a trauma. But, over time this can create dysfunctional habits, strong muscles get stronger and weak muscles get weaker. If we continue to move this way, it can become a bad habit. But it takes just one moment of awareness to change it. The moment you tell yourself "stop clenching my butt muscles when I stand in the grocery store line," you are now creating a new habit. A day will come where you check in with your butt muscles and find that they are relaxed.

The same can be said of being aware of how you feel when you eat or drink. The moment you bring awareness to how you feel after you drink a soda versus water, your awareness of what healthy feels like, shifts. That's how habits change.

Bring awareness of how you feel after you consistently stretch after a workout. Notice how you feel mentally and emotionally when you start the day with a positive affirmation and awareness. Being in the here and now, being aware of how your choices affect your mind, body, and spirit. Awareness is how you take an active role in your moment-to-moment health. This will lead to amazing changes and ultimately improve your quality of life.

Now: What Now? (No, Now.)

The concept is simple. You know that you cannot change the past and you do not control the future. Yet, that does not stop you from stress, worry, or guilt. If you pour those emotions into situations that you cannot change, they can have a negative effect on your health. Guilt, worry, and fear need a lot more energy than simply stopping, breathing, and allowing yourself to be in the moment. Letting go of things you cannot change. It's about getting out of your head and into your body. What is going on in your body, now, is the only truth that matters. It is the only moment where you can affect change.

Once you commit to making consistent, healthy choices through awareness of the here and now, you are taking essential steps. Each moment that you make the choice to be mindfully present, you are healthy, whole, and happy. You are all that you need to be. You are who you are meant to be, in that moment.

Is being mindful 100% of the time the goal? No way! That's not realistic. The point is to create goals that are easily achievable. So, taking one moment at a time is the only goal. We have all stepped out of our car once we arrived at home and realized, "Wow, I don't remember much of the drive here." Not remembering how you got somewhere is proof that you were not present in the moment. Our day-to-day tasks become so routine that we could do it in our sleep. Accessing the now could not be any simpler. In fact, we were given the very best tool at birth: it is called the breath. We will further explore this amazing tool later in the book.

Grow: How Do I Grow, Let Alone Be Grateful and Let Go?

Once we begin to start applying daily awareness, it becomes easier to make consistent, healthy choices. Then we can let go of everything that does not apply. Self-doubt, worry, fear, and negative thinking are just a few of the pieces that we can let go of. Once your arms have let go of everything you do not need to hold onto—such as fear and worry—they are free to pull in that which you do need—such as self-love, patience, and kindness.

Bringing gratitude and love of self and others is the only way to grow. Not letting go or failing to be grateful anchor us down to the same daily routines that contribute to unhealthy habits and choices. And too often, that anchor is our friend; the one consistent thing in our lives, and letting it go can be scary.

Remember that perfection is not the goal here. You will step off the path at times but making the pledge to commit to a daily healthy lifestyle is where it starts. Balancing fun, healthy eating, exercising, family time, and working hard with passion and zeal become more natural. And you will be so much more aware of how it feels once you stray. The scales will tip.

Elimination diets follow this same concept. Once you eliminate a food that you might be sensitive to, such as dairy, you might not immediately notice the positive effects on your mood and energy. Eat that food again after a month or so, and most people say that they can immediately feel a difference. Now you are motivated to continue to grow and let go. You have experienced what true health feels like. You are proud of yourself. You have experienced success. You feel better about yourself and this will reflect throughout your life.

So, try the same with positive thinking. Challenge yourself to be aware of one negative or judgmental statement that you make to yourself daily. Whether it's, "Ugh, I'm fat," "I don't look good in this," "I hate my hair," or "I'm so disorganized," pick one statement and commit to changing it to a positive statement every day. Your positive outlook will grow.

I have read articles and talked with people who have lived long lives and couples who have successful marriages or partnerships of fifty years or more. "Avoid negative people and situations" seems to be a very common theme from these successful couples and people. It is quite impossible to grow in an environment that does not support your growth and happiness. A solid foundation is essential from which to grow and live a vibrant life. You are building upon your selfcare matrix with consistent, healthy choices. Moment-to-moment awareness now allows you to let go that which is holding you back. Once you are free from that anchor, fly free, my friend. From a place of growth and gratitude, the possibilities are endless. Empowerment of yourself and others is now assured.

Empowerment: What is it and How Do I Get It?

Dictionary.com defines "empower" as; 1. give (someone) the authority or power to do something, and 2. make (someone) stronger and more confident, especially in controlling their life and claiming their rights.[10]

Commit to consistent, healthy choices through awareness of this moment. Being grateful and letting go automatically grow empowerment. Making the commitment towards selfcare is empowerment. Being an empowered consumer of your healthcare is what the core values of CHANGE are all about.

"To give someone the authority or power to do something" regarding your health and wellness is to put a lot of trust and faith in that person. As a health practitioner, I appreciate the amount of faith and trust my patients put in my team and me. Healthcare professionals should earn that trust. Providing individual, compassionate, quality care is the first step. But you, the patient, need to be included when planning your own treatment and goal setting. Your healthcare providers should encourage open communication every step of the way. It's your life and health that is at stake, not theirs.

It is your goals, and your definition of what "quality of life" means, not theirs. You are the team leader. We should hold each member of your healthcare team to this gold standard. Regardless of whether this is your healthcare team, recovery team, or friendship team, you need to set the boundaries and standards. You get to choose whether to stay in negative situations or relationships. It is your choice to eat foods that make you feel good and move in ways that allow you to function optimally. You make those decisions based on the CHANGE principles. Make consistent, healthy choices through awareness of the now. Allow yourself to grow and CHANGE. Those experiences introduce you to your body and how it feels, thinks, and functions. Make decisions based on that daily education. That is empowerment.

Empowerment has amazing side effects. Feeling good about yourself, empowered in your decisions, and present in the moment, makes you grateful for the journey. This, I believe, is at that heart of charity, of doing good things for others, helping them grow, and empowering them. Mother Teresa said, "Do not wait for leaders; do it alone, person to person. Be faithful in small things because it is in them that strength lies." I like to believe that by "small things" she meant everything from one person at a time to all the positive attributes of life. Health, happiness, trust, change, and the power of a smile are powerful small things.

Sharing the wealth of knowledge that you have gained on your health and wellness journey is how you can empower others. And never forget to give yourself a pat on the back, every day, for being you. Nobody can do that better than you! You now have a solid foundation from which to grow and CHANGE within the Selfcare Matrix.

Try This: Daily Change Check-In

Use the CHANGE values as the foundation to your selfcare habit decision making.

Is it something that makes you consistently feel healthy based on self-awareness whenever you check in here and now, moment by moment? Will it help you grow forward? Does it leave you feeling grateful and empowered?

C: Were you Consistent with at least one goal today?

   Yes   No

H: Did you make a Healthy choice today?

   Yes   No

A: Did you "check in" with Awareness what your body needs today?

   Yes   No

N: Did you stop to just sigh/breathe and be in the Now today?

   Yes   No

G: Did you take a step forward (Grow) with your goals today?

   Yes   No

E: Did you do something just for yourself today?

   Yes   No

E: Where you Empowered and make your needs known today?

   Yes   No

E: Did you set boundaries in order to achieve your goals today?

   Yes   No

PRINCIPLE #4:

LEARN TO HEAR

---

*"The most important thing in communication
is hearing what isn't said."*

—Peter Drucker

*Attention! These next three chapters are what will make the
difference in successfully applying the matrix to your life. They
will show you how to truly apply CHANGE with educated,
intelligent understanding of how your body works.*

Your Selfcare Matrix

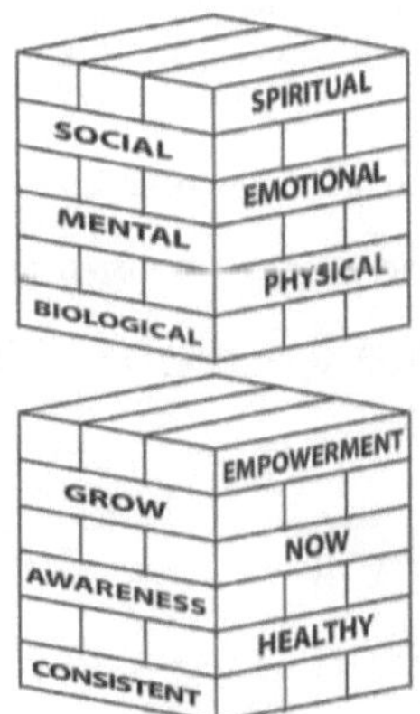

+ the whole you

Me, a Superhero?

"Mom, it hurts when I do this."
Mom: "Well, stop doing that." (Duh…)

Sound familiar? Common sense, right? You know this rule applies to others, but we so often do not apply it to our own lives. Yes, I "hear" my body tell me it hurts when I do this, but I do it anyway. We give into excuses such as "I'm just getting old." Your body is always talking; sometimes it whispers and sometimes it screams. All day long, our bodies give us signals. It tells us that we are tired, hungry, uncomfortable, hurting, scared, anxious, sad, and so on. Pain is most likely the one signal that can be the loudest. But somewhere along the way, we have learned that pain is something to be ignored and endured, not heard and attended to. In therapy, "I have a high pain tolerance" really means "I have a lot of practice ignoring my pain".

Today, stress levels are higher than ever. Sedentary lifestyles are also becoming more the norm within our personal and professional lives. If you have an active job, chances are that you often perform the same movement repeatedly. This is called "repetitive strain" and can lead to repetitive use injury such as carpal tunnel syndrome, tennis elbow or knee pain. These three things combined: high levels of consistent daily stress, sedentary jobs, and repetitive movements over the years, are likened to three villains in a superhero action movie. Your body is the superhero.

The human body's ability to change and heal is one of the most amazing things on this planet. It deserves the title of superhero. But if it is repeatedly hit by our leading villains, well, you might as well bathe Superman in kryptonite.

And true to superhero stories, you—our hero—have been leading a normal, boring life, having no idea that your superhero powers are lying dormant deep within you. What will awaken these powers? Why, a disturbance in the force, of course! But tapping into the force is the real trick. That power is always there and always has been. Can't you hear it? I know what you are thinking; "Ok, great, I'm a superhero, whatever. How do I hear this force that is supposedly within me?"

What is Hearing versus Listening?

"Hearing" simply refers to being aware of subtle changes in the atmosphere. For the purposes of this conversation, the atmosphere is your body. Hearing is your awareness.

"Listening" refers to acting. Hearing is more passive and listening more active. Listening is acting upon your awareness of your whole-body needs.

You are sitting in a park reading. You actually "hear" a lot of different and constant sounds such as birds singing, traffic buzzing, and a baby crying. But it is not until you stop reading, pay active attention or awareness to the sound that your brain then labels that sound as a bird singing or baby crying. You then think, "I didn't bring a baby with me today, so it's not my problem."

You can choose to ignore what you are hearing and put your awareness and energy back into comprehending what you are reading. You still hear the birds and the baby, but your awareness is on the book. That is your choice. You go back to reading your book, but the baby keeps crying.

You decide that you can't ignore it any longer. It is affecting your ability to focus on your book. You now take action to understand the meaning of what you hear. You are now listening. You decide how closely you want to listen. How much more information do you want? You can choose to leave the park to get away from the crying, or you can investigate the sound. You stop reading and shift your awareness to the source of the sound. You begin to understand what it means by getting more detail. How far away is the baby? Is anyone with the baby? Do you need to check on the baby?

When it comes to your selfcare, I am not only referring to the actual "using of your ears" kind of hearing. I am referring to the "awareness of all of the sensations within in your body" type of hearing. This really requires all your senses. "Hearing" is more passive than "listening." It is simply a perception or awareness that there has been a disturbance in the atmosphere as "sound waves," or your body's signals, hit your ears. Yet, when it comes to improving selfcare, the "atmosphere" is within your body – the sound waves can be any subtle change in whatever you consider normal in your daily bodily function.

Going throughout your day typically, you say, "I feel good," i.e. you're not hungry or in pain. Yet, when your stomach "rumbles," it sometimes can be heard and sometimes felt. But it should not be rumbling or gurgling all the time. You should not be aware of every part of your body all the time, how exhausting would that be? So, we "hear" this disturbance in the environment of our body as something different. You can hear it, "Oh, my stomach is gurgling," and make the choice to ignore it and go back to what you were doing. Or choose to stop what you were doing and say to yourself, "My stomach is gurgling. When was the last time I ate? Four hours ago! I must be hungry." Then you go eat. That is listening—acting based on what you "heard." Hearing your body's signals and taking the appropriate action is selfcare.

Sounds easy, right? Common sense, right? Yet, to "hear," you must check in with your body. How often do you stop what you are doing and simply "check in" with how your body is feeling? I'm sure you relate to this scenario. "I have to pee, but I need to finish vacuuming. Two hours later, you go to the bathroom, because if you don't, you'll pee your pants—if you haven't already. Typically, it is only when your body is screaming so loudly that you can no longer ignore it.

Therapy is another typical example. People do not seek out PT or OT if they are able to do everything they need to do. It's only when injury or illness absolutely stops you from doing the things that you want to do, that you finally seek help. Aside from our annual physical exams, we do not seek medical attention unless our bodies are screaming loudly. Or unless the illness or injury has been going on so long that your quality of life has taken a nosedive. If I had a nickel every time a person told me that they "just woke up" with shoulder (or back, or neck, etc.) pain, I'd be a wealthy woman. For when I ask them "Really? Have you never noticed that pain ever before?" After thinking about it and getting more history, they usually say, "Oh yeah, well, once in third grade, and another time in college..."

So, before you can hear your body's signals, be it whispers or screams, you have to be aware. And how do you become aware? Yes, you must be present, in the here and now. You need conscious awareness of your body's signals before you can ever determine what it means and then you need to know how or what to do with that information.

We are all aware of what it feels like to have 'butterflies' in our stomach. That signal can mean everything from feeling scared, nervous, excited, happy, or terrified. Or maybe we just have to poop. We also feel gut instincts, but how many of us act on them? Trust them? Hearing your body's signals is to first connect that feeling with a specific area of the body. To do that, you must first take the time to hear the signal. You then have to trust it enough that you are willing to listen. Then you need to have a healthcare team that you trust will hear, listen and help you translate the body's signals. Only then can you make a successful selfcare plan.

A beautiful example of ignoring your body's signals is how common dehydration can be in the elderly population. In the general population as well. Research suggests that one in five older people living in long-term care homes do not drink enough fluid."[11] Drinking less water can be a result of a diminished sense of thirst. The more we ignore the subtle signals of thirst, often misunderstood as hunger, the more dehydrated we become. In another study, "Following water deprivation older persons are less thirsty and drink less fluid compared to younger person…when dehydrated older persons are offered a highly palatable selection of drinks, this also failed to result in an increased fluid intake."[28] The more dehydrated we become, the more subtle the sense of thirst can become.

The more you ignore your body's signals, the harder it is to effectively "hear" what your body is saying. You ignore your body's signals enough, it stops talking. It learns the only way to get attention is to break down. Consistent selfcare aims to avoid that.

How Does a Whole-Body Health Approach Help Me?

A solid understanding of the body is essential before you can learn to hear and then interpret what these signals mean. This is the important "know-why" part of the learning before we get to the "know-how." An "integrative approach" to health is not only integrating a team of like-minded people with different sets of skills, "integrated" also refers to how we should approach our own selfcare. To "integrate," or bring together that which is separate, is essential if we are to better hear, listen and respond to our body's needs. Everything in our body is connected or "integrated." The more you and your team understands that, the more effective the Selfcare Matrix will be.

Often, more subtle signals should be addressed immediately. Prevention of injury depends on our willingness to act on the subtle messages. Injury is often not felt until our bodies start "screaming."

Think of a child gently tugging on your shirt, "Mom I need you." If you are in the middle of something—as we so often are—you might not stop what you are doing and listen to the child's needs. Then the child starts yanking on our shirt, jumping up and down and screaming, "Mom I have to pee!" By that time, it might be too late. Now you have an accident to clean up. If only you had heard and acted the first time!

To combine the components that make you uniquely human, you need to understand that you are not just your physical body. In yoga, the body is further divided into bodies or dimensions. Throughout the years I have adapted the concept of "bodies" and teach it as an inter-connection of systems. You are a combination of everything that makes you wholly you.

My professional experience has taught me the benefit of treating the body as a whole, integrated system. The ultimate goal of an OT or PT should be their patient being independently able to maintain his or her progress. Which means teaching the person how everything is connected.

I Have Six Systems?

Even though you are one whole you, it is easier to understand if I break it down into six systems. I like to use the five bodies or categories from my yoga background. I have added another body or system that I'll refer to as "biological." I am discussing them as separate "systems." Yet, understand that just as your mind and body are not separate, these systems must work together. These systems make up one body, you.

In healthcare, all medical professionals are broken up into specialties and subspecialties. The body (or the combination of our systems—see chart below), is so incredibly complex. There is no way to truly understand it all—or be an expert—without breaking it down into parts. There are psychologists, internal medicine physicians, neurologists, orthopedic surgeons, urologists, gastroenterologists, gynecologists, optometrists, massage therapists, physical and occupational therapists—you get the idea.

But you are not just your body or just your mind. The saying "It's all in your head" has a negative connotation. When told by a doctor that it is "all in your head," or "psychological," or "just anxiety," the takeaway message tends to be that it's not real or that you are making it up. You are a hopeless case. It is a phrase often tagged onto a patient that cannot be diagnosed with objective and measurable scientific data, such as with blood work or an MRI. I am speaking from experience when I say it does nothing to positively contribute to your health. It can feel like the mental equivalent of being smacked in the face and told to leave and not come back.

Guess what? Yes, it is "in your head," or "psychological!" Everything is "psychological." A basic definition of psychology is the study of how the mind works in relation to how it affects behavior. To simplify it, your brain is in your head. How you perceive pain is in your head. You don't perceive pain in your body but in your brain and spinal cord. There is constant research trying to better understand chronic pain. We are just starting to understand how all the systems interact when pain is in the body for a long time. Terms such as psychobiological, cognitive, emotional and behavioral are being used to show how all the systems interact.[30] How you behave, or act, comes from the interaction of the complicated network of how all the different "systems" in your body interacts. But if you were just a brain, how would you hug your family, or run, or live and grow. All the systems working together are what it means to be human. To interact, to grow, to learn, be quiet and loud and active and peaceful, contemplative and wild.

To be a "healthy" human is to have a balanced interaction of all of our "systems." So, let's stop thinking of our body's systems as separate. Instead, let us see how all six of the systems integrate with each other and ultimately make "you" you. This is important to understand if we are ever going to hear, let alone know, what the heck to do once we've "heard" what your body has to say.

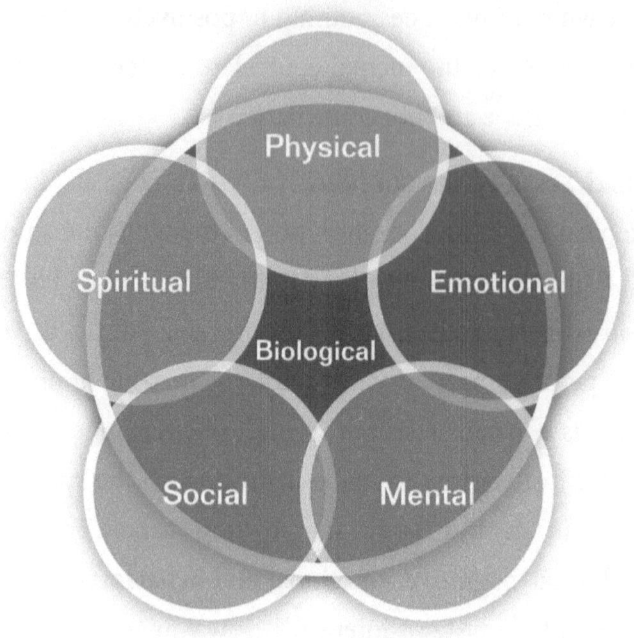

Six Systems of Whole Body Health

Biological System: My Biology is a Sticky Situation?

I have separated "biological" health from "physical" health. This is based on my observations and what I have learned as an occupational therapist treating chronic pain. Dealing with Lyme has only solidified my clinical reasoning on the matter.

We will dive further into the "biological" system in the next chapter. Stick with me, it gets complicated. But you are worth the time and effort it will take to help you better understand. The better you understand yourself, the better you will help your healthcare team help you.

I do want to mention that within this system is another "matrix," called the "extracellular matrix." "This is living tissue within the body and can be thought of as a dynamic meshwork of cells and liquid. Despite their close proximity to each other, the cells of a tissue are not simply tightly wound together. Instead, they are spaced out with the help of the extracellular meshwork."[12] And this "stuff" is everywhere. It is one of the reasons why we say everything in the body is connected. It connects, or sticks, everything, to everywhere. This network of tissue creates the spaces for all the other tissues from all the other organs to weave through.

In Thomas Meyers book "Anatomy Trains," he quotes Dr. James Oschman: "…the extracellar matrix is a continuous and dynamic "supermolecular" webwork extending into every nook and cranny of the body; a nuclear matrix within a cellular matrix within a connective tissue matrix. In essence when you touch a human body, you are touching an intimately connected system composed of virtually all the molecules within the body linked together."[57] An amazing spider-work network all available with your every move.

When our physical bodies are stuck in the same positions or movement patterns these tissues can get stuck too. This can stop or disrupt the flow of fluid that is essential for whole body health. This is one of the reasons why professional massage and manual tissue work is so important when healing. Exercising and stretching alone is not enough.

Physical System: Why Should I Just Keep Swimming?

According to one study, there are an estimated 23.4 million adults (10.3 percent) experiencing high levels of pain, and an estimated 126 million adults (55.7 percent) reported "some type of pain" in the three months prior to the survey.[13] That's a lot of people. Yet, most often you would not know who is living with chronic pain by looking at them. Many of them are "functioning." They work, drive, and take care of their families.

Physically, they look just fine. Ask anyone with chronic health issues how it feels when someone tells him or her, "But you look so good" or "You don't look sick." Yes, physically we function, our bones, joints and muscles still function, and we can live life. But it is their quality of life that matters. If the more you move the more you hurt or burn up your limited energy because, "biologically" you are not stable, then your quality of life is affected.

The physical system tends to be the only system we ever think of when it comes to health. If you can't move because of pain or fatigue, you seek help. If you can't swim, you drown. This system refers to what you can see, touch, and feel. It is your "house" or your "temple," so take care of it. Your physical system refers to your skin, joints, muscles, and tissues. It is interconnected with your biological and all other systems. There are four types of tissues, muscles being one of them. The other three are the nerves, skin, and organs.

Connective tissue is present throughout your entire body and systems. It supports other tissues and binds them together, including bone and lymph tissues, as well as the tissues that give support and structure to the skin and internal organs. The health of these tissues is essential to posture and movement. The health of connective tissue is dependent on blood and fluid flow. Moving in many different ways—shortening and lengthening—is essential for the health of your physical system.

Whether you deal with arthritis, constipation, or fibromyalgia, movement is so important. Physical movement, such as jumping, walking, and waving your arms, pumps your fluids to all your parts. This is necessary for survival. Aging affects our living tissue health. It affects every body differently. But aging is not an excuse to not let your health go. Balanced movement is important for physical and biological health at every age.[14]

There are always ways to move no matter your state of health. Dory, the loveable and forgetful character in Pixar's "Finding Nemo," likes to say, "just keep swimming." I find it helpful to remember to that when I am less motivated. Just move.

Mental System: Feeling Nervous?

By now you should begin to see how the matrix is never-ending, dynamic, and inter-connected. It is not whole without each part. Notice how all the systems interact with each other? The same systems serve many different functions within many different systems.

Mental health is directly linked to your overall health. Mental health refers to the function of your brain. Your brain and spinal cord make up your nervous system, which is the ultimate super hero in your personal health story. It is the interaction of the brain and spinal cord that can determine how well you deal with pain. And research shows that thinking something is happening, such as you are about to be attacked, can actually have physical effects on the body.[31] Your mental, emotional, and physical bodies are very intertwined.

Your entire system was created to survive as a hunter and gatherer living in the woods. This means that your nervous system is designed for fight or flight—be on the ready to fight for your survival or to run away, instead of being eaten by a tiger or an enemy tribe. Though most of us are no longer running for our lives from a tribe or animal trying to eat us, our nervous system still interprets daily stress the same way. When your body thinks you are in danger, some systems "amp up" and others slow down. Your mental and emotional states are directly linked to your physical system. So, when your mind senses a reason to fear and protect, your physical body is immediately ready to react. And you now know that our daily fears are not about getting eaten by tigers but being late for work. But your body reacts the same, no matter the fear.

So, you are walking in the woods, gathering berries to feed your tribal family, and all your senses are on the alert. Your vision and hearing are more aware. You hear a rustle in the leaves, which could mean danger, and your body prepares to flee. Your head and shoulders move forward, your muscles tense. Your heart rate and breathing increase. The blood flows to the center of your body because this will be more effective to help you run away. Your sympathetic nervous system—fight or flight— prepares you for survival. This is called the "cascade defense." Animals have the same defensive response but "unlike animals, which generally are able to restore their standard mode of functioning once the danger is past, humans often are not, and they may find themselves locked into the same, recurring pattern of response tied in with the original danger or trauma."[32] Understanding our mind-body patterns to these responses—which become rote and involuntary—is very important for developing treatment interventions and a selfcare plan.

When you feel scared or stressed, it is not time to relax, pee, or poop.

Your parasympathetic nervous system controls the body's "rest and digest" functions. In times of stress, organs such as the intestines and bladder slow down to focus on the more important task: survival. Blood flow goes to the "flight" organs, such as your heart and muscles. This is teamwork at its finest. Except most of us are not hunters and gatherers any more. We are not in constant danger and do not need to be on that level of alertness all the time. Yet, we often are under a constant state of pressure and that often goes hand in hand with stress.

I refer to it as "sympathetic distress." When you are constantly worrying about what you did do, did not do, or still have to do, you are living in the past or future, rather than being in the here and now—in this present moment. Our nervous systems function the same way as if we were in constant danger. This is exhausting to all our systems. It can lead to the breakdown of one part of a system, or even entire systems. For example, if you are constantly worrying about things you can't control and there is never a solution, the worry continues. Your body is constantly prepared to flee. Therefore, the body doesn't have time to relax, pee, or poop.

What happens to your digestion? It slows down. Your body is learning that it must "hold it" all of the time. What do we call this? Constipation. Four million people in the United States have frequent constipation. It's the most common digestive complaint.[15]

So yes, mental health and digestion affect each other; not to mention sleep, heart health, appetite, and sex drive. This brings me back to the fact that people blame these issues on psychology. Mental and emotional health is essential for physical health. Pain is perceived in the brain via chemical reactions and affects your physical body's function. Your brain's health is your mental health and therefore your physical health—they are connected; there is no separation. They all need to be addressed together if you are going to experience any long-lasting change.

Quieting down the mind and hearing your body's signals leads to listening. So, understanding where in the body you are sensing, or hearing messages, requires a basic understanding of how the organs, tissues, and emotions affect each other. Where in your body do you feel or hear things? The fancy term for this is "somatovisceral." "Soma" refers to the sensations of the organs, combined with the sensations or awareness of the muscles and joints. It is essentially how muscles, nerves and ligaments "cross-talk" with organs and can be why heart attack symptoms can be perceived and felt in completely different areas of the body from person to person.[16]

Thus, somatovisceral is your awareness in space combined with the awareness of what your body is feeling on the inside. Checking in with this helps you better understand the whole picture of your body. With the sense of touch, from your skin, we get sensations such as temperature or pain. Your visceral—or organ—sensation gives you a deeper awareness of your internal state, such as a feeling of fullness, shortness of breath, or a racing heart. This sensory system is just another of many amazing systems set in place to help with your survival, health and healing. The goal is not to control or worry about everything in your body, just to be aware. Education, and improving your sensation and awareness of your body is the starting point.[17, 18]

The goal is not to control, or worry about, everything in your body, but just to be aware.

Emotional System: My Body Has A Map?

Your emotional system prepares you to meet daily challenges by adjusting how your body's systems interact, including your heart, muscles and bones, brain, nerves, and hormones. The way you speak of your emotions every day proves this link; "I have a gut feeling" or "I was heartbroken" or "I have cold feet," or "I have butterflies in my stomach."

Let's look at a study, called "Bodily Maps of Emotions." It explores how our emotional states affect our bodies. It shows how our bodies can physically react to certain emotions. This then affects how we behave in certain situations. Several similarities were found across cultures. I find it fascinating and have definitely noted the same sensations in my body.

People were asked to map on a body outline where in their bodies they feel emotions. Warm colors represented where they felt an increase in sensation and cooler colors a decrease. They found universal similarities. The positive emotions (happiness, love, and pride) formed one cluster, whereas negative emotions split into four clusters (anger and fear; anxiety and shame; sadness and depression; and disgust, contempt, and envy). Surprise—neither a negative nor a positive emotion—belonged to the last cluster, the neutral emotional state remained distinct from all other categories. They found several similarities in where we feel or perceive emotions in very specific areas of our bodies.[19]

(See Chart Below AFTER doing the TRY THIS exercise.)

Try This: My Emotions Map

Wherever you are, make yourself comfortable. Close your eyes and take your time imagining each scenario. Color in the areas on the blank body outlines exactly where in the body you are feeling each emotion. Do not question it, mark your very first sensation. Try making up some of your own scenarios. Use different colors for different emotions.

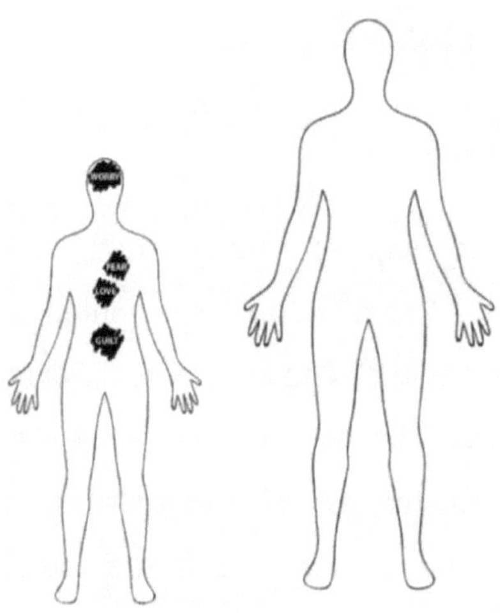

- *Fear: You are lost in the woods and it's getting dark. You do not have any way to get help and you do not have any food or water.*
- *Love: You are watching a romantic movie where the couple finally confesses their love.*
- *Excitement: You just found out that you are going to have a baby after years of trying.*

- *Frustration. You are having a bad day, and nothing's going right. When you go home, your child or partner asks for help, you yell, and they start crying or yelling back.*
- *Nervous. You are at the starting line of your first three-mile race.*

There is no right or wrong answer here. Your body is your body and where you feel and perceive emotions will be unique to you. Now compare your "emotional maps" with the study outcomes below.

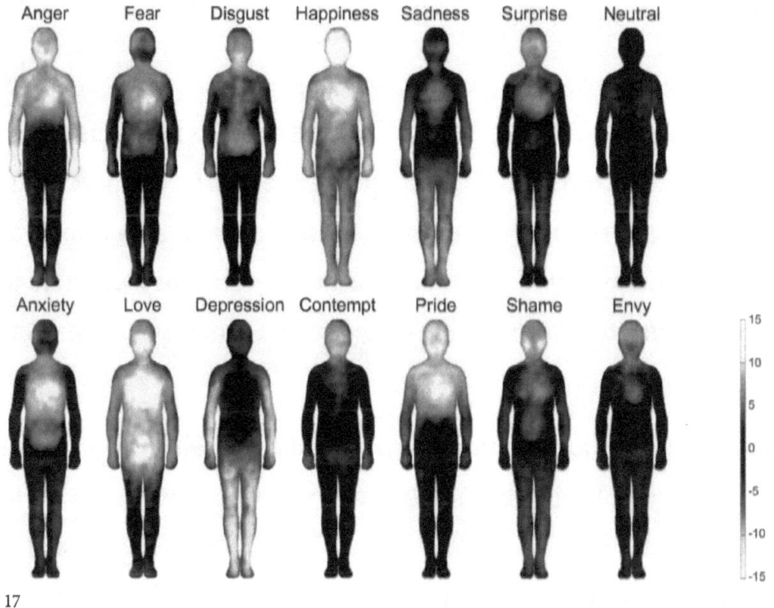

17

The above map is from the study mentioned earlier. It shows where in the body emotions tend to be felt in the body. Everybody is different, so it may differ for you. Hearing and then listening is so important, it shows how your body is speaking to you, all you need is to listen. Notice how love and happiness are felt almost throughout the entire body; yet depression and sadness leave the lower body void of warmth and blood flow.

Social System: We Need Each Other?

As you saw in the chart above, your social health is connected to your mental and emotional health. Social emotions, such as love and happiness, have global affects in the body. Lack of social health, depression and sadness, seem connected in where they are felt in the body. And speaking of connections, that is what your social health and well-being are all about. I am the kind of person who can make friends easily. Call me an extrovert, but I get so focused on my personal and professional goals that I rarely make the time to socialize.

As humans we are completely interdependent on each other. And somewhere along the line, we have learned that it is bad to ask for help or to rely on each other. That independence means doing everything by yourself, so you try to be everything to everyone. This mindset can suck your energy dry. Yet, taking time out of your busy schedule to sit and just chat with your spouse—as you did when you first met—is rejuvenating.

Enjoying each other's company—that is social health. Taking time to play can mean playing on a softball team, having coffee with a friend, or talking with your kids about their day at school. Being present with the people around you. And do I need to say that face-to-face connections need to be balanced with social media interactions? Connecting with people has many benefits. It contributes to your "whole body health" on every level of every system.

Spiritual System: Can You Say: "I Will Survive. I Will Not Give Up."

Spirituality means many things to many people. You will determine what spiritual health means for you. Here, I will refer to spirituality as defined by a model we use in occupational therapy, namely the Canadian Model of Human Occupation and Engagement (CMOP-E). This model places spirituality at the core of the person (that's you). It refers to spirituality as the main aspect of being. It is your source of will, self-determination, sense of meaning, and purpose. It is your sense of connectedness within every environment you enter.

Your spirituality or will and determination are the power behind achieving your selfcare or any goals. It may be your faith in God, nature or the human connection. This is the fire that keeps your Selfcare Matrix growing. Without a sense of hope, will, perseverance, and determination, you cannot achieve anything. You do not grow. Yes, self-doubt is always there. Depression, pain, fatigue, and anxiety can whisper in your ear, "You can't do that," "You're stupid, ugly, weird, and worthless." If you let that voice win, you no longer engage. Your sense of purpose in this life dwindles, making you ask, "Is it worth it?"

This is your core or essence – it is who you are and what is important to you. This system intertwines within every one of your systems. Therefore, the health of this system can make or break your whole-body health. Having a true sense of purpose—feeling empowered—is what makes everything else worth it. For some, God is the power behind their faith. For others, it is serving their community or simply being true to themselves. You get to decide. Ignoring this system and what it means for you, will set you up for failure.

What Does the Whole Me Sound Like?

To best understand what each system is, let us just explore. It is much easier to hear anything when you are in a quiet environment. And if you have ever tried to stop thinking, you know that it often feels impossible. I love the Buddhist concept of monkey mind. The monkey—or your ego—will constantly chatter in your mind. It plants self-doubt and stifles your creativity. But if you give the monkey a banana, he will stop chattering and focus on the banana. Taking slow, deep breaths is the banana you give to your monkey to quiet down your mind, saying, "Here, monkey, pay attention to this."[20]

Focusing on the breath is often the best way to get out of your head and into your body. Stop thinking and just breathe for a moment. This does several wonderful things for your entire body. To begin to hear, you first need to quiet down your environment, or your mind. Your mind is what will hear, or perceive, your body's signals. You need to be present within your own atmosphere. This is where selfcare begins.

TRY THIS: Four Exercises

1. Diaphragmatic breathing

No matter where you are, take a moment to close your eyes. Take a slow, deep breath in through your nostrils and out through your nostrils or relaxed lips. Try breathing in for a count of 2-3 and out for a count of 4-6. Feel the cool air flow into your nose and let the warm air flow out. Do this three times.

Open your eyes. What were you thinking about? Hopefully, nothing. You were probably just focusing on breathing. This is the space where you can begin to hear. When first learning, you will need a quiet external environment. Your bedroom works well, but eventually, you will be able to do this anywhere, anytime. With your eyes open or closed.

Check out my YouTube video on this technique:
Diaphragmatic Breathing!

https://www.youtube.com/watch?v=L5bRe28fCQA&feature=youtu.be

2. Map It Out

What did you feel? What did you hear? Was it pain somewhere in the body? Stiffness? Muscle tension, such as clenched fists or shoulders pulled up toward your ears? Is it a nervous feeling in your stomach? Do what feels right here. Write the word you feel in the body part, such as "pain" or "scared," a color that feels right, or pain number, 0 = no pain, 10 = extreme pain. Since we only did a few breaths, maybe you heard nothing. That's fine, move onto the next exercise.

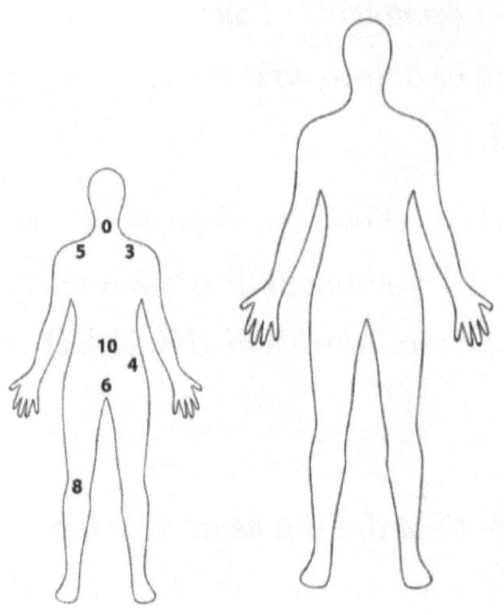

3. Interpret What You Hear

Continue to be aware of your slow breathing. Now, you are going to explore your comfort level in each of your six systems. There are no right or wrong answers; just check in and hear. Pretend you are a detective searching for signals that apply to each of your systems. You are looking for a comfort-level score.

On a scale of 0 to 10, how comfortable are you in each of the following areas? Zero equals complete and total comfort, happiness, a sense of relaxation, and no pain or discomfort noted. Ten is extreme discomfort. This area is screaming at you for attention.

- *Biological (B): After breathing three or four times, things should now be quiet within your environment. What is your state of health? Do you feel stuck? Do you fail to see improvement in your health no matter what you do? The first thought or answer is all you need. Hear it, then move on to the next system. It does not matter if you agree. Score 0 1 2 3 4 5 6 7 8 9 10*

- *Physical (P): After breathing 3 or 4 times, go to the first area you feel in your body. Right now, I get drawn to my right butt cheek as I'm sitting on this chair. Score 0 1 2 3 4 5 6 7 8 9 10*

- *Mental (M): Are you able to focus on the breathing, or are you very distracted? Does stopping to breathe and "checking in" feel impossible or do you hate these types of exercises? No judgment just listen. This will be heard or felt more in the mind. Score 0 1 2 3 4 5 6 7 8 9 10*

- *Emotional (E): This is typically heard or felt in the abdomen and/or heart region. What's the first feeling that comes to mind? No right or wrong answer; only objective observation; no personal opinions. This is self-awareness.*

- *Social (S): When you think of your relationships with others, how does it feel in your body? Where do you feel it in your body? Do you feel more tense, more relaxed, happy, or sad? Score 0 1 2 3 4 5 6 7 8 9 10*

- *Spiritual (SP): What feeling does this word or topic evoke in your body? Do you feel that you have a purpose on this earth? Do you have a sense of connection and support? How strong is your will and determination to improve your health and achieve your goals? Score 0 1 2 3 4 5 6 7 8 9 10*

4. Map It Out Again

Now write the letter in the area on the body where you heard each system; or, you can write the word corresponding to what you heard, such as "pain" or "scared" in the area of the body that you felt it, such as in the right arm or your heart.

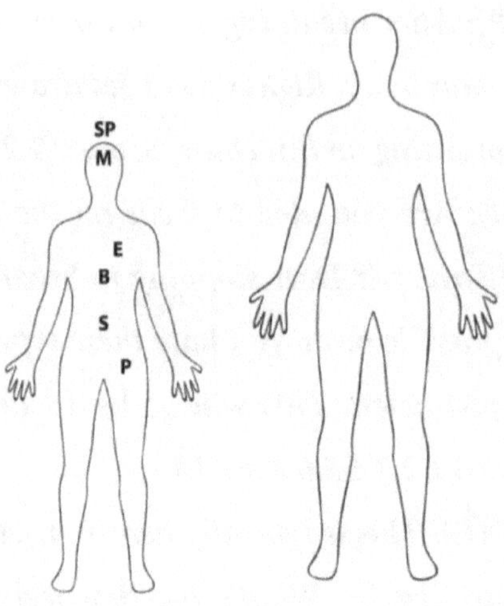

PRINCIPLE #5:

LEARNING TO LISTEN

"Your work is to discover your world and then with all your heart give yourself to it."

— *Buddha*

Your Selfcare Matrix

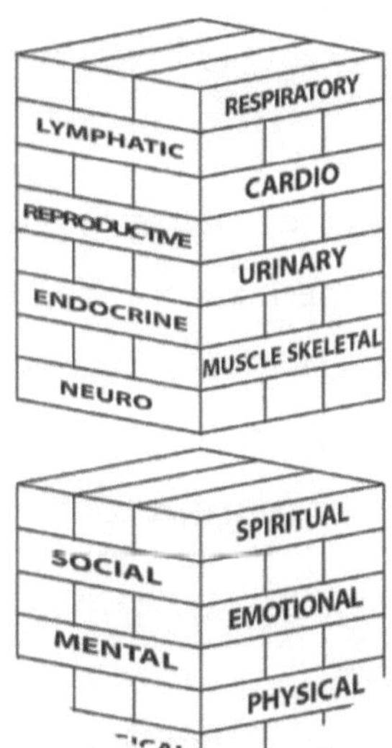

+ balanced biology

What Do I Do Now?

Your body welcomes you. You cannot change what you do not know. Now that you have practiced hearing, awareness is the key to better knowing and understanding. Listening creates awareness. You need awareness and understanding before you can act. Taking a few moments to hear and listen will change your life in so many ways. You've stopped to check in with your body and have scores based on what you have heard. You have moved from being disconnected to a state of reconnecting. Reconnecting every day will give you the power of awareness, acceptance, and change.

Welcome to your body! It has so much to tell you. And like reading a book, your own personal story offers many lessons to be learned.

Next comes the tricky part. It is time to translate what you hear into what it means for your health and well-being. What the heck does each signal mean?

First, know that you become better at what you practice. I love the phrase "practice makes permanent." So, the more you practice quieting the mind and hearing what it has to say, the easier it will be to respond—not react—in a way that helps you heal and grow as well as communicate with your health care team.

I am not necessarily saying that you have to learn to sit and meditate thirty minutes a day, every day, for the rest of your life. Will that be helpful to your health? Sure. But I want you to learn how to incorporate it into your day. This way you can hear and listen at any given moment and act accordingly. For example, sitting at your desk, you hear your back hurts, so you change positions. You no longer hear anything, so you go back to what you were doing—back pain diverted, yea, go you! You have to pee, but you just peed thirty minutes ago, so you stop to breathe or relax, check back in, and you no longer have to pee. Yea, look at you being in control!

Try This: Emotions Map

THIS IS A REIVEW OF OUR FIRST EXERCISE IN CHAPTER FOUR.

Wherever you are, get comfortable. Close your eyes and imagine each scenario. Using different colors or corresponding numbers, note where in the body you are feeling each situation:

1. *You are lost in the woods and it's getting dark. You do not have any way to get help and you do not have any food or water.*
2. *You are watching an incredibly moving, romantic movie where the couple finally confesses their love.*
3. *Your wife just told you that you are going to have a baby after years of trying.*
4. *You are having a bad day, and nothing's going right. When you go home, your child or partner asks for help, you yell, and they start crying or yelling back.*
5. *You are at the starting line of your first three mile race.*

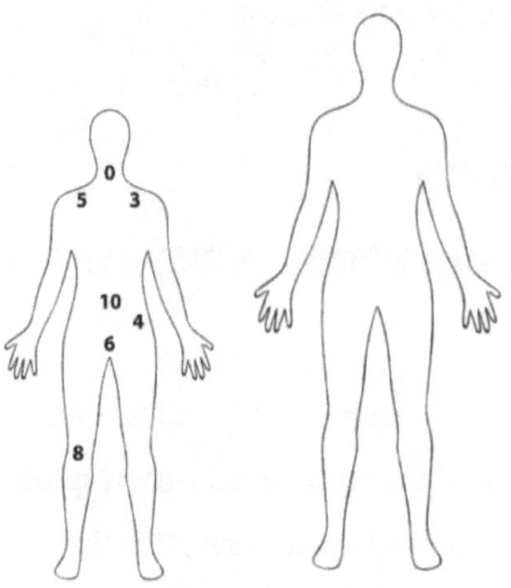

Why Should I Care About Balancing My Biology?

Now you are conscious and aware of the sensations in your body. Next, you must understand how to analyze what it means before you can understand what to do about it. Hold on, strap in and please stick with me here. I promise reading this will be worth it.

Let's begin with a basic understanding of the eleven systems within your physical body. This is what I refer to as the biological system. To simplify it, this system is made up of nerves, vessels, muscles, organs, fluids and other tissues that work together as an integrative team. When one or more of the systems fail—if we are not healthy on a cellular or biological level—then it's "Houston, we have a problem." In therapy, if you do not heal and progress toward your goals at a normal rate then you may have to go back to the drawing board; back to your healthcare team to assess your biological health. In this chapter, we will explore why biological health is at the heart of your whole-body health.

Can You Please Tell Me about the Basics?

Your organs function in more than one system and serve more than one function. You don't need to have a master's degree to understand the "basics" of human survival. Before you can hear, listen, and speak your body's needs, you first need a basic understanding of how a body works. Within your biological system you have eleven systems that must all function properly for you to be healthy and functioning properly in life. Let's explore them.

The 11 Systems of Your Biological Body

1.NEUROLOGICAL

2. DIGESTIVE

3. SKELETAL

4. MUSCULAR

5. INTEGUMENTARY (Skin, hair, nails)

6. ENDOCRINE

7. URINARY

8. REPRODUCTIVE

9. CARDIO (circulatory)

10. LYMPHATIC

11. RESPIRATORY

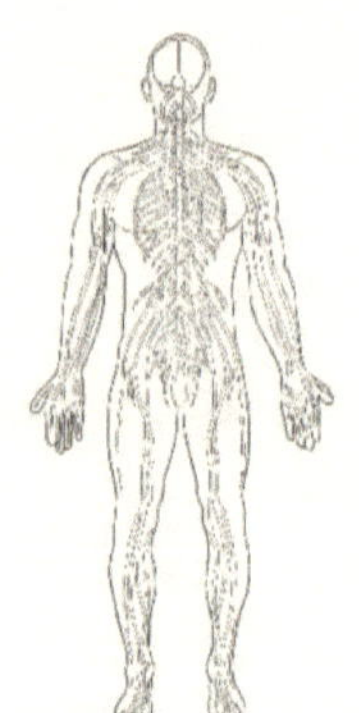

1. Neurological System

Nervous (neurological) system: Brain, spinal cord and nerves. Pain perception, emotion, thought, and rapid response to the environment.

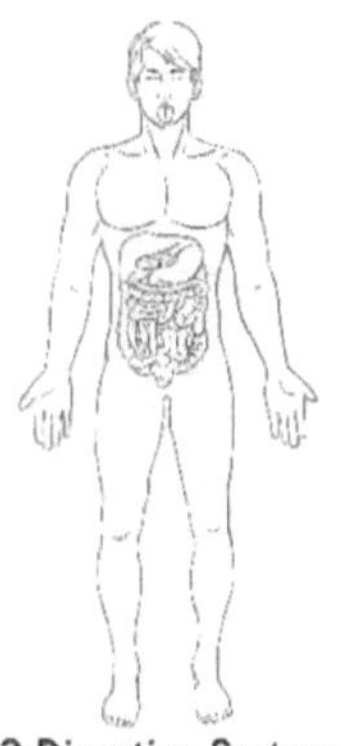

2.Digestive System

Digestive system: Mouth, stomach, esophagus intestines, gallbladder, liver, has its own enteric nervous system. (Think: mouth to rectum and everything in between.) About 70% of your immune system is in your gut. Gut health is SUPER important to your overall health.

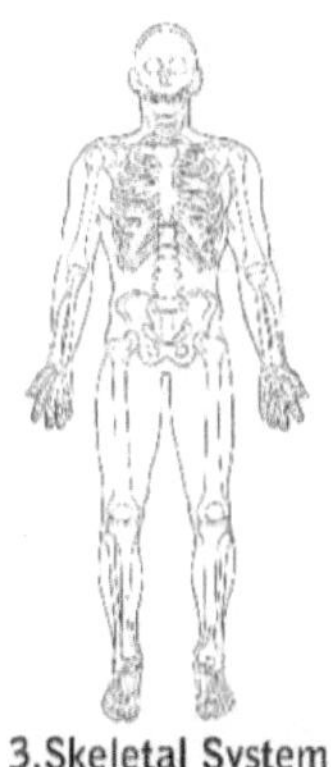
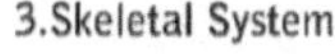

3.Skeletal System

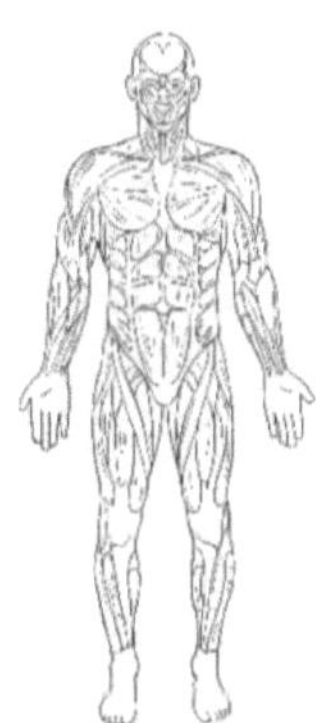

4.Muscular System

Musculoskeletal system: Muscles, connective tissues and bones (I am combining the muscular and skeletal systems)—moves the body—from walking, squatting, feeding, hugging, running, fighting. Muscles and bones.

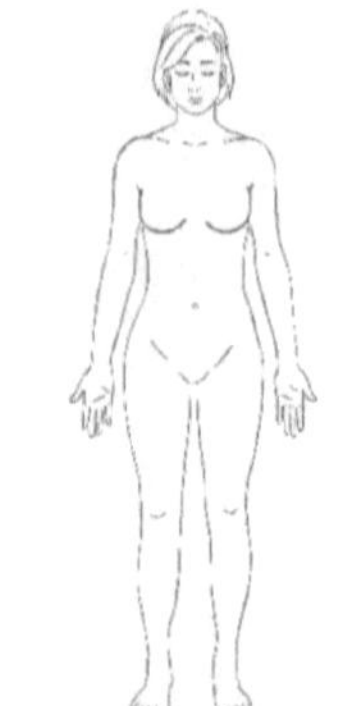

5.Integumentary System

Integumentary (skin) system: Skin, hair, nails, sweat and other glands, and nerves. Its main function is to act as a barrier. It protects the body from the outside world. It also functions to retain body fluids, protect against disease, eliminate waste products, and regulate body temperature.[35]

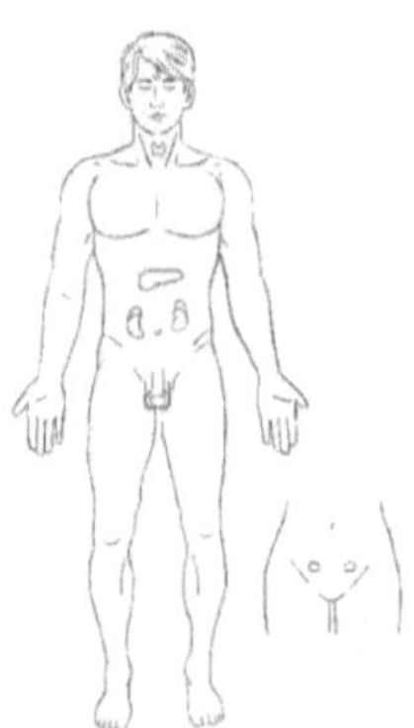

6.Endocrine System

Endocrine (Hormones) system: Pineal and pituitary gland in the brain; the thyroid gland, adrenal glands, pancreas, ovaries and testes. The endocrine system is not well understood amongst the public, but SUPER important to your health.

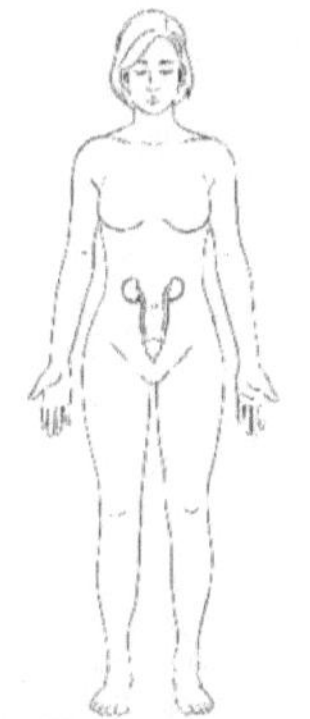

7.Urinary System

Urinary/Renal system: Kidneys, bladder, ureters, and urethra. Produces, stores, moves and eliminates fluids called urine. The kidneys make urine by filtering extra water from the blood and any other waste. The kidneys move the urine through the ureters to the bladder and out the urethra. "Extra water" is key here so drink your water, people!

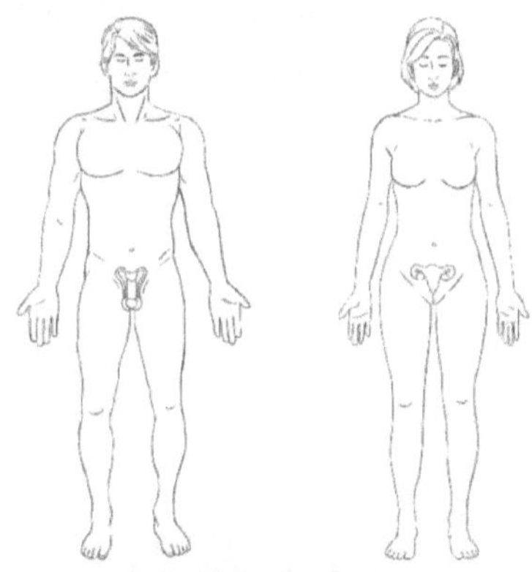

8.Reproductive System

Reproductive system: Male: Includes the penis, scrotum, testes, sperm and a series of ducts, fluids and glands. Women: Includes ovaries, fallopian tubes, uterus, vagina, vulva, mammary glands and breasts. The organs in both the male and female are involved in the production and transportation of gametes and the production of sex hormones. The goal of this system is the fertilization of the egg by sperm to start and support the development of offspring during pregnancy and infancy.[55]

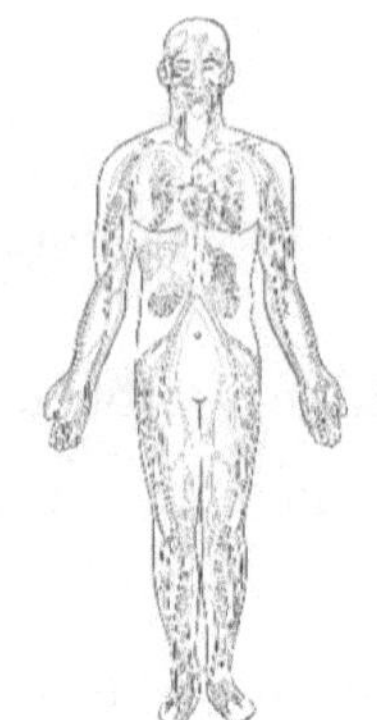

9.Cardiovascular System

Cardiovascular system (Circulatory): Heart, arteries, veins, (think neck, chest and upper back and arms region) Moves materials between different body systems including oxygen, hormones, nutrients and waste.

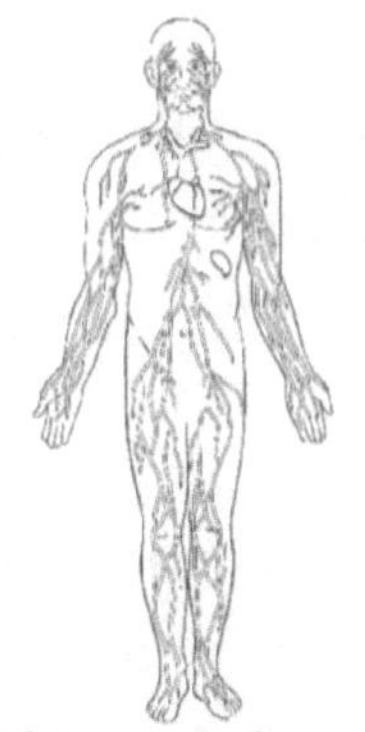

10.Lymphatic System

Lymphatic/Immune system: Lymphatic vessels and nodes permeate the body. (Think: entire body, head to feet, but heavily concentrated in armpits and groin.) This system is intertwined with your digestive system.

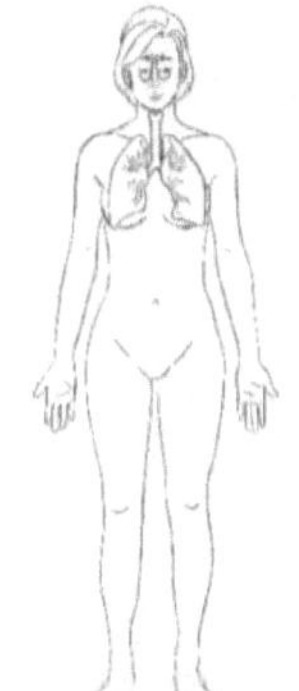

11.Respiratory System

Respiratory system: Gas exchange between your cells and the environment. Delivers oxygen to your blood and removes carbon dioxide (and gives it to the trees). It also acts as the pressure system and regulator in the body. One way the upper half of your body is connected to your lower half.

95

How Do I Survive?

To stay alive, you must have basic biological health. These systems support your life. When these systems stop working, severe illness occurs and death can follow. They are the foundation on which your whole-body health depends.[21, 22]

Abraham Maslow was an American psychologist and was an advocate of viewing people in terms of what motivated them, instead of seeing them as a "bag of symptoms."[34] He researched elite college students and exemplary people, such as Albert Einstein. Following the study, he developed "Maslow's Hierarchy of Needs," which has five distinct groups. To achieve happiness, we first must satisfy our physiological, or most basic needs first. This is the basis of the pyramid in his model (see below).

If your most basic health needs are not met, you are stuck in survival mode, such as a furiously busy mind. You may feel as if you have no space in your life, you're stressed, tense and hyper-reactive.[33] Being stuck in survival mode prevents us from having any leftover energy to do anything more complex in life, such as working, exercising, or having quality time with our kids.[34] Your biology needs to be healthy and in balance. Only then can you free up your ability to focus on what matters most rather than focusing on things that don't matter, such as TV, addictions, or compulsions due to frustration and stress. Selfcare starts with kindness and self-honesty, which we know now how to achieve with our new-found hearing and listening skills. Honesty then begins the process of building up our foundation: starting from our biology to feel sane and alive. Your biology functions well, you feel great, your mind is clear. You can focus on what is most important to you like having loving relationships or climbing Mount Everest.[33]

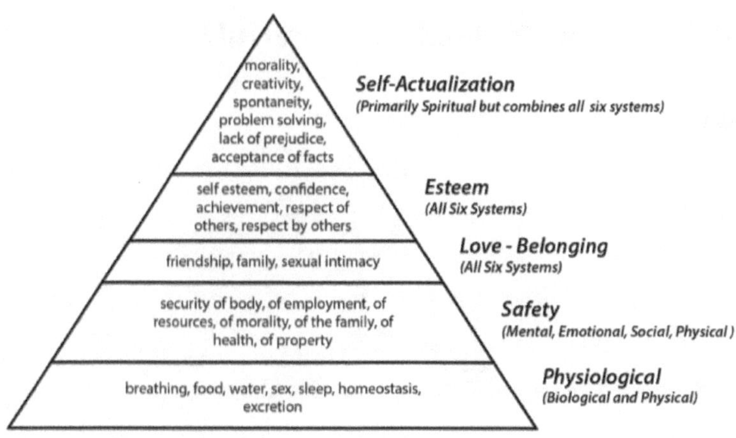

Malow's Hierarchy of Needs and the Whole-Body Health Systems

Our Most Basic Needs for Survival or Core Fundamental Needs[34, 33]

- Moving/Reacting ("Homeostasis," or living in biological balance, also known as "not dying")
- Eating/Drinking
- Reproducing
- Socializing/Community
- Breathing
- Peeing and Pooping
- Sleeping

Below you will see how the eleven biological systems all interact to perform the foundational needs for our survival. It is amazing to see how they are all connected. Since we have established that the health of these systems is the foundation for your whole-body health, you see why biological health is such a high selfcare priority. Later in the book we will discuss how to address the health of these systems.

What Are My Basic Needs for Survival?

<u>Moving</u>

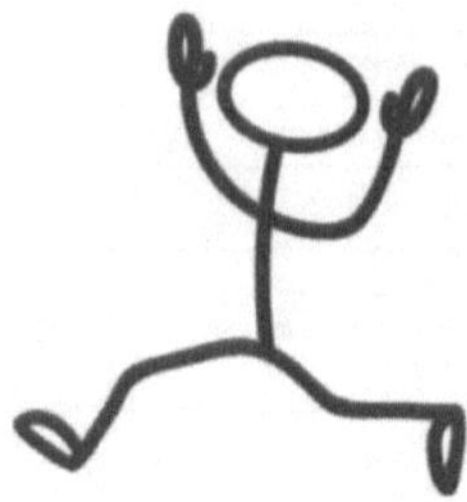

Fight or Flight: Allows you to be alert, adaptable, and flexible to respond to the environment.

How Everything Connects: The **nervous system** is how we communicate with the outside world. It is also the command center for many functions inside our body. It processes our sensations to triggers reactions, such as making you move or feel pain. It is through the two part of the nervous system that then communicate the need to use your other systems such as your **muscle** and **skeletal system** to run or react quickly to changes, and your **skin, hormones, heart** and **lymphatic system** to sweat and then cool your body down again.[50] Sexual arousal (**reproductive system**) is also part of fight or flight.

<u>**Sleeping**</u>

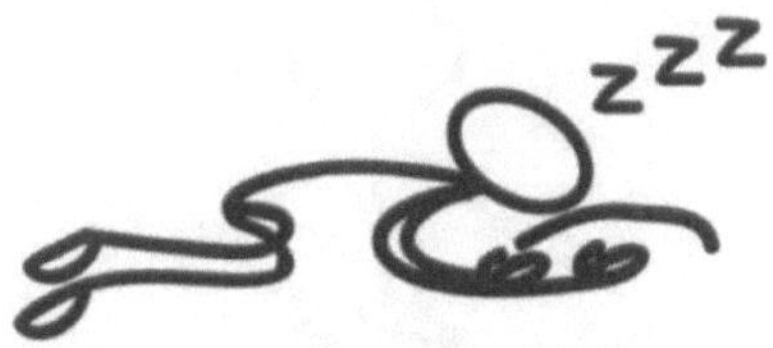

Rest and Digest: Opposite of moving or "fight and flight." It allows the body to rest and the organs to re-group for such as bowel, bladder, and heart. This is essential for it allows you to be alert, adaptable, and flexible to respond to the environment. If you are not rested, you are not as alert when awake and need to function.

How Everything Connects: In addition to heart, circulatory, digestion and urinary system health sleep is essential for the health of all your other systems too. Deep **sleep** triggers **the** body to release hormones that aid in normal growth in children and teens, boosts **muscle** mass and helps repair cells. **Sleep** also plays a role in puberty and fertility. **Your** immune **system** relies on **sleep** to stay healthy.[49]

<u>**Breathing**</u>

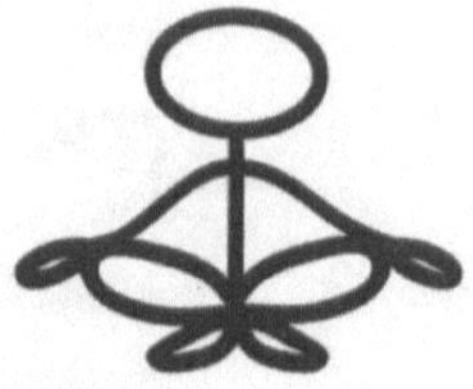

Just Breathe: Being able to take in oxygen and release carbon dioxide (excrete waste) for biological (cell) health.

How Everything Connects: Besides the obvious function of breathing (respiratory system) it also affects movement control, postural stability (**muscle** and **bones**), and plays many important roles in your physical and psychological health. It can also help your body keep itself in balance by influencing the nervous, **heart, skin, lymphatic, endocrine, digestive** and **urinary systems.**[51]

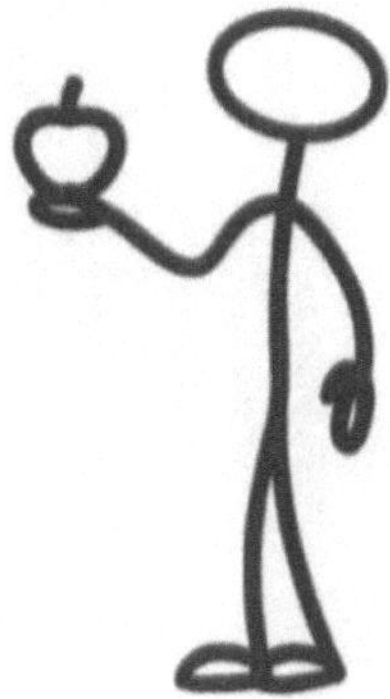

To Ingest or Not to Ingest: Taking in (food in), and release/digest, (waste out), to deliver proper nutrients to your cells.

How Everything Connects: Your body needs nutrients from food and drink to work properly and be healthy. The nutrients from water keep every system in your body healthy especially your skin, tissues (**muscles, bones**, and organs involved in your **cardio, digestive, reproductive** and **urinary systems**). The nutrients from food and water help with the circulation or movement and distribution of fluids, chemicals and hormones Your **digestive** system further uses the breaks nutrients from eating and drinking into parts small enough for your body to absorb and use for energy (**nervous**), growth (**reproductive**), and cell repair (**lymphatic, respiratory, endocrine**).[52]

<u>**Peeing and Pooping**</u>

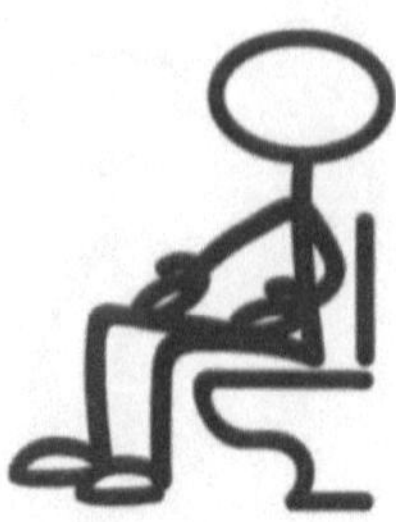

Move It Through, Keep What You Need and Get Rid of the Rest: Being able to clear toxic waste products from the body.

How Everything Connects: The **nervous system** is very involved here. The nerves tell certain **muscles** when to tense and when to relax. Nerves in the spinal cord send messages from the brain to the bladder. Sphincter muscles control the flow of urine, for your **urinary system**. Muscles in the rectum and anus control or release stool for your **digestive system.**[53] Besides filtering and eliminating wastes from the body, the urinary system also maintains the balance of water, ions, pH, blood pressure and calcium via the kidneys and other organs and tissues. Therefore, the **lymphatic, heart, skin, respiratory** and **endocrine** systems are also involved.[54]

<u>**Socializing**</u>

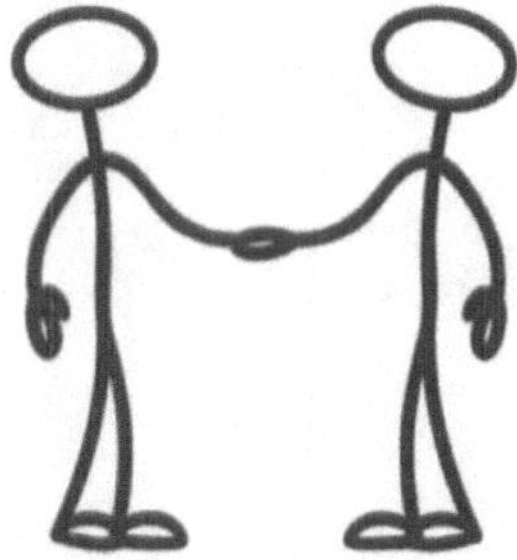

Interaction Within and Without: Okay, you might have to stretch your imagination a little here. But "socializing" here means not only our need for a sense of community on the outside but also within your body as well. think about what you need to interact with others.

How Everything Connects: Our bodies need to be healthy and able to interact within and without. Our **skin** and **lymphatic systems** are important to fight infections, secrete hormones, and protect the body's organs from the environment. All necessary aspects of surviving and socializing. Our **circulatory** and **endocrine** systems affect secretion of hormone which are chemical substances produced in the body that regulate the activity of cells or organs. They regulate the body's growth, metabolism (the physical and chemical processes of the body), and sexual development and function, also a part of "socializing." So, all other systems are used here as well: **nervous, musculoskeletal, respiratory, reproductive, digestive,** and **urinary**.

<u>**Reproducing**</u>

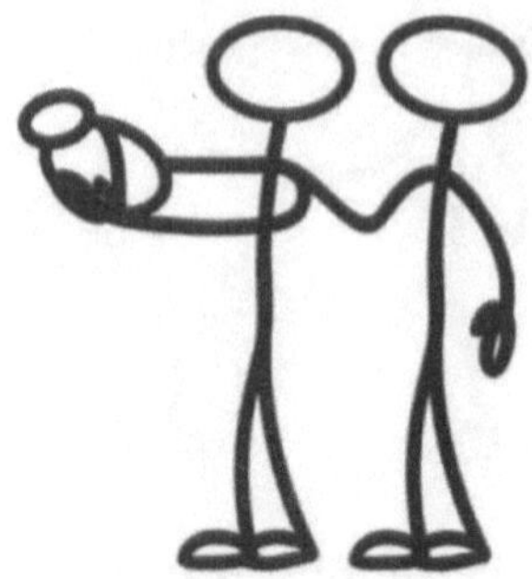

Making Whoopee: Having sex/make babies/reproduce: Very necessary for a species to survive. It must be able to reproduce.

How Everything Connects: Reproduction is dependent on hormone production. This is a very complicated subject and all systems can be affected by lack of balanced hormones, at any age. Men need to produce sperm and women eggs to make a baby. The **nervous system** is involved in arousal which then affects the **heart, musculoskeletal, skin, respiratory** and **lymphatic system** as tissues, glands and fluid flow are involved in erection and ejaculation. The **endocrine system** produces hormone which are essential for the growth of a fetus and is a lifelong balancing act. The **digestive** and **urinary systems** need to respond to the nervous system properly for everything to function properly.

Try This: Putting it All Together

Using a word or color, mark where in your body you feel the following scenarios:

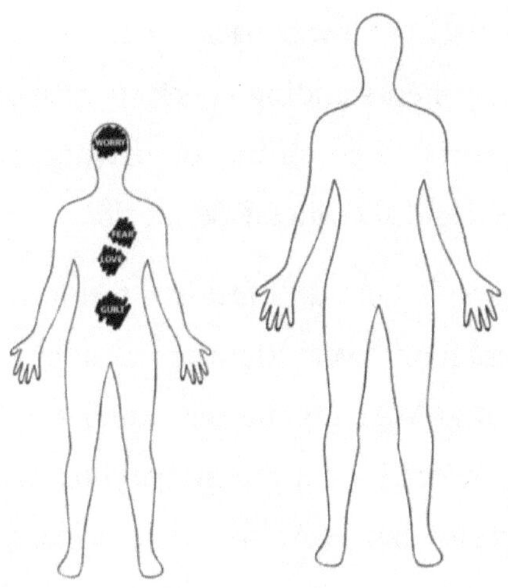

- *Fight with your spouse*
- *"Don't feel good"*
- *Feel the urge to poop*
- *After you exercise*
- *Didn't drink water all day*
- *Sat in a meeting or classroom for several hours*
- *Have to talk in front of a group of people. Before, during, and after?*
- *Meeting with a close friend that you haven't seen in a while*
- *Ate greasy food*

Come up with a list of scenarios where you know you can create pain, tension, or discomfort. Maybe you always hurt sitting at work, or perhaps you avoid going out in public or talking to someone because you feel nervous. Where do you feel fear, exhaustion, or excitement?

Now that you stopped to hear, you will get drawn to a particular body part or area of the body. Listen, and then act. My back hurts standing like this, so I change position. Did that help? Maybe, you feel pain in your spine, upper back or lower back, or in between your shoulder blades. Be specific. When standing check in with your butt muscles. Can you relax them? When sitting or driving, can you let go of tension in your neck and shoulders? Be specific.

I feel tired and angry. Where do I feel it? I feel it in my stomach. Is it in my upper abdomen or lower? Right or left side? Is it pain, tightness, stretching or bloating? When is the last time I ate? Four hours ago. I eat. How do I feel now? I ate a greasy hamburger. How do I feel? I drank water and ate a salad. How does that feel versus how I feel after I ate the hamburger?

Go back and compare with your body outlines from the Chapter 4: Exercise 2 and 4 with the last two exercises from this chapter. You may notice commonalities with where you feel emotions and basic needs. You may or may not be surprised with where you are consistently noting muscle tension or pain. Are you seeing connections between where you feel basic needs, muscle tension and pain with different emotions? Remember, every system is connected so that constant right shoulder tension may be connected to that nervous feeling or stressed sensation in your right stomach or belly area. Constant anxiety or worry can put constant strain on your heart or digestive system. Pair this with not eating right or not exercising regularly and you could have a recipe for disaster.

You will be amazed at how much checking in and creating awareness of how you feel throughout the day will help you understand what your body is trying to tell you. It is constantly talking to you; you only need to listen. The more you listen, the more you learn. The more you learn, the more motivated you will be to take care of yourself. The more you do for yourself, the easier it will be to communicate with those around you, those who want to help you reach your whole health potential. Your healthcare team and your friends and family are your support team—your circle of trust.

Congrats, you just performed selfcare. You're playing a proactive role in caring for your overall health and well-being. Take a few moments throughout your day to notice what you feel in your body. Try it before and after you do something such as eating, sitting in a meeting, hiking, or fighting with a spouse. Checking-in will give you a better understanding of what actions and attitudes contribute to your health and what depletes your health. Then, and only then, can you make conscious decisions about your selfcare and health care. You cannot control what happens around you most of the time. Stress will always happen, but you can decide what to do about it and so be responsible for your actions.

How Do I Calm it All Down?

You should be so proud of yourself! You have taken the time to learn how to slow down, hear and listen to what and where your body is trying to communicate with you. Showing your body that you will take the time to listen and act is the only way to create change in how your body reacts. If every time you feel stressed your body reacts by tensioning muscles in your butt or belly, it will always do that unless you tell it otherwise. Change the habit, create a new one.

I liken it to training a puppy. If, for the past 10 years your "puppy" has walked at your side nipping at your heel, you allow it by ignoring it, he will always do it. Then one day you look down and say, "Stop it," he will stop, look at you, and go back to nipping at your heel. But if you continue to train him, stop a couple of times throughout the day to check in and tell him "no," eventually you will go to check-in and notice that he is just walking, calmly, next to you. You have taught him a new habit.

Taking the time to stop and check in will you help you create new, healthy habits. Learning to calm and balance your nervous and muscle systems will have a very positive affect on your other nine biological systems and is therefore a great place to start. And, most importantly, there are several easy ways to do it.

Try this: Progressive Relaxation

Now that we have messed with your emotions and learned how your body responds, try this easy technique. Check in and release any tension or discomfort that we may have stirred up.

https://www.youtube.com/watch?v=h6JLkGn1UYk&feature=youtu.be

Lie down or find the most comfortable position for you. Take a moment to check in with your comfort level scale as we did earlier. On a scale of 0 to 10, how comfortable are you in your own skin right now? "Zero" means completely chill, 10 means extremely uncomfortable/tense, whether it means pain or anxiousness, it's your call.

Then, take a few slow, deep breaths, and just settle into your body. The emphasis in the exercise is to feel the difference between muscle tension and relaxation. So really draw out the exhale. Take time to feel the exhale. Feel the muscles melting, relaxing. We want to create a new "baseline" of normal. Release the muscle tension and note how you feel in your body afterwards.

Bring your awareness down to your feet. At the same time inhale and tighten every part of your feet and toes. Squeeze your toes, point your toes, or pull them up toward your face. Exhale and release the tension. Next, inhale and tense your legs as tightly as possible, then exhale and feel them melt/relax back down in to the bed or chair.

Next, inhale, squeeze your butt cheeks together, and exhale as you let them melt back down. Inhale and tense your belly and chest muscles as tightly as you can, then exhale and melt them down.

Inhale. Tense the muscles of your hands and arms. Keep your shoulders either very straight or curled into your body. Exhale and release. Inhale as you tense your shoulders up toward your neck. Exhale and release. Inhale and tense the muscles in your face and tongue. Exhale and release.

Lastly, inhale and tense your entire body. If you want to scream, tense the muscle of your throat as well, and let it all out with a nice, big sigh. Now release, relax everything, and trust the support of your bed or chair.

Take a few more slow, deep breaths. Check back in and score your comfort level. Has it changed? How? Where in your body has it changed? How can you incorporate this technique throughout your day?

Do You Loathe Looking in the Mirror?

Truly hearing and listening to your body means now you have awareness. Awareness of your body's moment-by-moment signals as well as what it might possibly mean. The more you listen the more you'll hear. The more you act the more your body will trust your actions. You will hear more "thirst" signals, and better understand thirst versus hunger signals. You'll be more trusting of when the signals mean go to the emergency room or call your doctor. You are now accountable for your actions.

If you are now aware that eating fast food makes you feel sluggish and depletes your energy, then so what? You can choose to eat it anyway because darn it, you love pizza. Now that you are choosing out of a state of awareness, you accept the consequences.

I have patients that come to therapy with complaints of bladder leakage. Journaling a few days of their eating, drinking, and peeing habits can be enlightening. And very often, we see a connection between what they drink and urgency—a strong sense of needing to pee.

Urgency and leakage can go hand in hand. For many, it is after several cups of coffee, alcohol, or even certain foods. Finding what foods or fluids lead to leakage is an awesome discovery. I call it "holding the mirror up to your day." Looking at your habits, in your physical body or your behaviors, is so empowering as it brings an understanding as to what can contribute to urgency, leakage, or pain. None of this is normal and should not be accepted as such! Once you have an awareness of what contributes to your symptoms, now you have choices. You get to decide when – and whether—to drink or eat whatever it is that causes the urgency and leakage, or not. You are learning how to control your habits instead of feeling like your body, in the case of urgency, your bladder, is controlling you. How liberating! This is empowerment, my gift to you.

If you find coffee contributes to leakage, now you have a choice. You love coffee, you can decide if it's worth it to possibly leak in public. You—not your bladder—decide to wear a pad when you go have coffee with your friends. You have back pain whenever you sit in your favorite chair. Now you are aware of the cause of your pain, you have a choice; replace it or limit the amount of time you will sit in it. Pain and leakage are two very motivating symptoms. They can encourage us to change our habits. But wouldn't it be nice to stop it, either before it happens, or before it gets so out of control that it takes over your life? For this to happen, you will need to step out of your comfort zone. Do the unthinkable: talk about your problems and ask for help.

PRINCIPLE #6:

LEARNING TO SPEAK

"If you don't go after what you want, you'll never have it. If you don't ask, the answer is always no. If you don't step forward, you're always in the same place."

— *Nora Roberts*

Your Selfcare Matrix

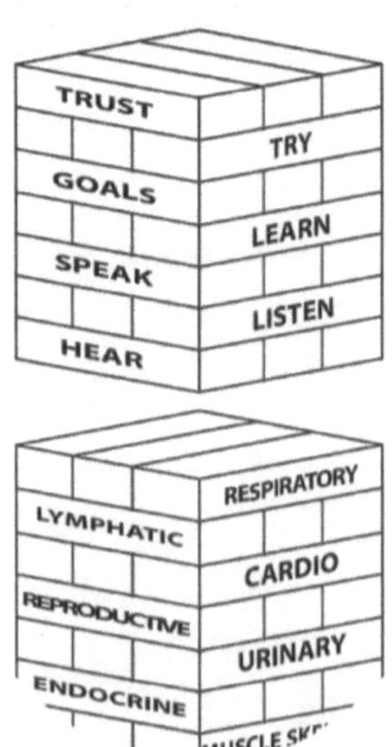

+ colossal communication

Who is the #1 Expert about Me?

Working in small outpatient clinics, therapists are often expected to meet with doctors to educate them about our unique services. This was terrifying to me. I know a lot of people feel intimidated by doctors whether speaking to them as a colleague or as a patient. I was very intimidated by their amount of knowledge and was sure that I would look stupid and inept. Who was I to think that I could teach a doctor anything? But the more I stepped out of my comfort zone, and talked to them, the more I was able to see him/her as a human that was an expert in A field of science, and not MY field.

There are so many different fields of study when it comes to understanding and treating the human body, that it is impossible to know it all. That is why there are so many specialties in healthcare, such as urology, physical therapy, internal medicine, oncology, etc. Imagine how many "fields" of land there are on this planet. A farmer tending to his or her piece of land, no matter how big, will know their land better than anyone else does. But they would need to be taught, educated, how to tend to any other piece of land. This principle holds true for medical professionals, too. An orthopedic surgeon will have a better understanding of how a joint should work than an oncologist, for example.

What I want you to understand, is that NO ONE knows your body better than you do. Yes, your internal medicine doctor (or primary care physician), has a better overall understanding of human anatomy, physiology, and biological health than you do. But if you speak to them from a place of daily awareness you will be the ideal patient. Only you know how it feels when you sit at a desk all day, if your sex drive is "normal" compared to two years ago, what position feels best to sleep in, or how your body reacts to stress or a specific medication.

Only you know what makes you feel happy, sad, or excited. Only you know what it feels like to be in your skin every day. So, you are the most important member of your healthcare team, because it is YOUR BODY and you know it best. You are the expert when it comes to your own body. But only if you listen and only if you speak up and communicate.

Colossal Communication: What, When, How and Why?

"The single biggest problem in communication
is the illusion that it has taken place."

— *George Bernard Shaw*

Success begins and ends with communication. The word "colossal" basically means "huge." It is so important to communicate your needs, thoughts, feelings, concerns, and ideas. It really is the gold-standard for any healthy relationship, namely the one between you and your complicated self. Communicating your needs should expand throughout your universe; mind, body, team, co-workers, friends, and family.

If you don't ask, they won't tell. One staggering statistic that I learned in pelvic floor therapy is that it takes a woman an average of six years to talk to their doctor about any issue going on "down there." Many of us think the word vagina or penis should be whispered.

My daughter was put in time-out in kindergarten for saying the word "butt" and her teacher had to whisper that word into my ear when explaining why she put my daughter in timeout. When did talking about our body become shameful?

If you are to put selfcare back into your daily priorities and make it the foundation of your healthcare, then you will need to speak up. Speak up about everything, especially the things you don't want to talk about. Just like mom always said, "the foods you hate are the ones you should eat because they are good for you." The same goes for what you'd rather not talk about.

The more you practice hearing and listening, the easier it will be to communicate what and where you feel things. Only then will your trusted medical team be able to better help you translate, understand, and guide you towards your options regarding what next steps to take.

Self-respect and clear communication are a two-way street. Now that you are practicing first hearing and then listening to your own body, you have a better understanding of how to hear and listen to others. Selfcare and self-respect go hand-in-hand. When you go to speak to your healthcare team member, be prepared to represent your needs from a place of self-respect and honor. Doing that will allow you to also be respectful of them as a human being—and as an expert in their field—which leads to gratitude. Being thankful to have them on your team means that you are open to what they have to say as well as having a willingness to consider and try their suggestions.

A Never-Ending Story?

Yes, it's one of my favorite movies and I'm not ashamed to admit it. And if you have seen it, you know that it is adventure-filled with lots of triumph and excitement. A boy and his horse team up with many different creatures. Like any good story, his journey allows him to cross paths with, and be-friend, creatures with unique and special skills. These skills help him complete his mission while narrowly escaping death. His ultimate goal is saving the world, only to lose all of his friends along the way. Oh, and the world blows apart into a million pieces. And yet, every part of the adventure—the sadness and loss, the bravery and excitement— all lead to the main character having a better understanding and respect of who he is and how his strengths and limitations make him unique. He learns that he could never have saved the world by himself.

Trusting in himself and others. Communicating his needs to both himself and his trusted team allowed him to see his power was always there, within him. But, if he hadn't trusted and communicated along the way, the "nothingness" would have prevailed and destroyed the world.

Yes, that is an extreme example. Ok, not communicating your needs and not trusting your bodies' signals may not end in world disaster but it is essential for the health and healing of your world, your body. Communicating, speaking clearly, and stating your needs is another essential step toward effective, daily selfcare. This communication is a continuous, never-ending cycle. This is the next layer in your Selfcare Matrix. Clear communication is based on what you "hear" your body is telling you. As a manager and business owner, I use these seven steps toward clear communication. These are your essential steps toward communicating with yourself and others.[23]

What are the 7 Steps Towards Clear Communication?

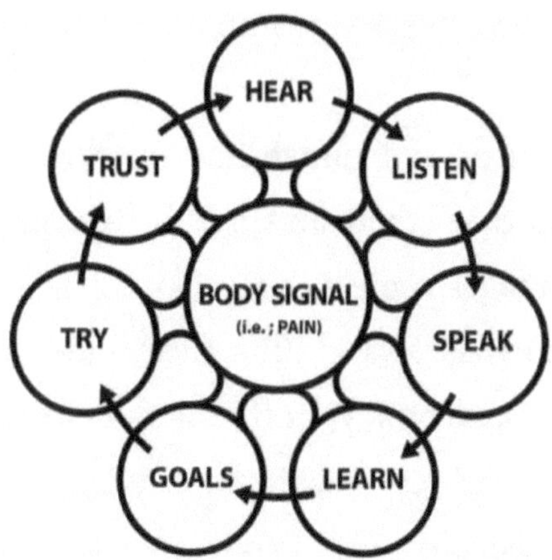

No matter where you start on the 7 steps cycle of communication just take it one step at a time. Speak or ask, then just listen and be silent. This step is so important and can often help you get more out of a conversation than when you do all of the talking. If you know what specifically you want to accomplish at your next healthcare team appointment, refer to the Guide Book for a version to fill out and bring with you. dnichols@motivatetherapy.com

- ❏ **SPEAK/ASK** Be clear about what your message is:
  - ❏ What do you want your team to understand?
  - ❏ What do you want to walk away with? What is making your goal for the appointment?
- ❏ **HEAR and LISTEN** Two-Way Street—Are you all eye contact? Are you clearly stating what you wanted to tell them? Do you understand what they are telling you? What are they not saying?
- ❏ **LEARN** Does it make sense? What other resources do they recommend? What do you want to learn at this appointment?

- ❑ **GOALS** Do you understand what they are saying? What goals are you agreeing upon? Do your goals differ? Make clear what your goals are, this is very important to communicate to your team.

- ❑ **TRY** If you do not understand or if you have tried and it hasn't helped, tell them and give them a chance to explain in a way that makes sense to you. Do not fear "looking stupid." Unless you walk away with a clear understanding of what is being suggested, both your time and theirs is wasted.

- ❑ **TRUST** You're responsible for any failure to communicate. This is selfcare 101. You are 100% responsible for understanding what is being said, in a way that contributes to your health and well-being. You both need to trust that open and honest communication is happening.

- ❑ What other questions do you have along the way? Write them down ahead of time and have a place to write down more questions during your appointment.

- ❑ **HEAR** Are you hearing them? Are they hearing you? Hearing and listening apply to your body as well as to interacting with others

- ❑ Repeat, Repeat, Repeat.

- ❑ Do not be afraid to say, "This is what I am hearing you say. Is that correct?" If it is not something you agree with, then repeat your needs until you both come up with a solution that is acceptable to you. Your body, your decision.

- ❑ Respect them, and they will respect you. Yes, when you visit your healthcare team member, the conversation is about you and your needs. But you need to be respectful of the other person, because they have certain goals to achieve as well. You must both believe in the message and the solution. You must respect where that person is coming from and sincerely care about the healthcare team's unique perspective. You are both taking time to be together and to listen to each other. Be respectful that you each have different motivations, areas of expertise, and needs.

*Clarify the message and solution that you
are hearing before leaving your appointment.*

❑ Did you ASK what you wanted based on what you are HEARING your body needs? Did you LISTEN in a way that you LEARNED what you set out to learn, and in a way that you feel confident to TRY what was suggested? Are you able to set GOALS for yourself based on clear communication? Did you feel comfortable communicating your needs? Is this person now a part of your CIRCLE OF TRUST?

Try This: Key Questions for Self:

Refer to the Guide Book for a version to fill out and hang somewhere visible to you every day.

- *What will I practice today? How can I communicate this to others?*
- *How will I deal with my body's signals today?*
- *Can I be accepting of how I deal with others at any given moment? Learning vs. judging my moment-by-moment reactions?*

- *How will I deal with conflict in a healthy way for me? And for others?*
- *What will I allow in? What will I let go of? How does it feel?*
- *What do I enjoy doing? What makes me happy? How can I do those things more often?*
- *I feel good in my (heart, body, stomach) when I (hang with friends, go for a hike, work with children).*
- *I feel bad in my (gut, neck, stomach) when I (yell at my kids, go to work).*

I love the saying "be an objective observer." Answer honestly and look back at your answers as though you were reading a friend's answers. Do not judge your answers; just know them as your truth at this moment in time. They can change every day.

Maybe pick a question that you will ask yourself every day before you get out of bed, to bring awareness to what you will practice that day. Beginning your day with awareness of how you feel will allow you to communicate your needs from moment to moment. If you say to yourself, "I will practice being happy today," you may be able to stop yourself participating in a conversation at work that does not contribute to your happiness. Saying, "Today I will practice being healthy" may help you make a healthy choice at lunch, or at least make you aware of the fact that it is a healthy choice—or not. You get to decide from moment to moment; accept it as a conscious decision and move on.

*Be confident in yourself and take ownership
for your decisions from a place of awareness.*

Try This: Report Card: A general question checklist for you to fill out prior to any appointment. This may help you get the most out of your appointment.

Check the ones that you know you will want to ask. Refer to the Guide Book for a version to fill out and bring with you to your next healthcare team appointment.

Now you will be better prepared to clearly speak your concerns and convey your needs to your healthcare team.

Report Card:

- ❑ *SPEAK/ASK: I feel (this) when I do (that). It doesn't go away. What can this mean?*

  ____

  ____

- ❑ *Pain Level: Currently (when you are at rest): _______/10*
    - ❑ *Best: ______/10 What makes it better?*
    - ❑ *Worse_________/10 What makes it worse?*

- ❑ *Other Symptoms I am worried about:*

  ____

  ____

- ❑ *LISTEN: What are my choices?*

  ____

  ____

❏ *Are there other choices?*

____

____

❏ *I don't feel comfortable with trying medication first. Are there other options?*

____

____

❏ *My insurance only covers:*

____

____

____

____

Are there other options?

____

____

❏ *LEARN: What are the consequences if I do not choose what you are suggesting as my first option? What can I do to learn more?*

____

____

____

❏   *GOALS: These are my goals:*

____

____

What can I do to meet them? Feel better? Get stronger? What have you done personally to improve your health? What have you seen work well with your patients in similar situations/diagnoses?

____

____

❏   *TRY: I read about this___________. What are your thoughts about this? What facts do you have about this subject? What do you suggest I read? What resources do you trust?*

____

____

❏   *TRUST: I have heard good things about (this PT, surgeon, massage therapist, or gym). What are your thoughts?*

____

____

❏   *If I'd like a second opinion, do you have any suggestions, resources?*

____

____

Find what works for you. Listen and trust your gut. This way you will feel more confident listening and trusting others. You get to choose your "circle of trust" and health care team.

DISCOVER AND DIRECT YOUR DREAM TEAM

"Coming together is a beginning. Keeping together is progress. Staying together is success."

— *Henry Ford*

Your Selfcare Matrix

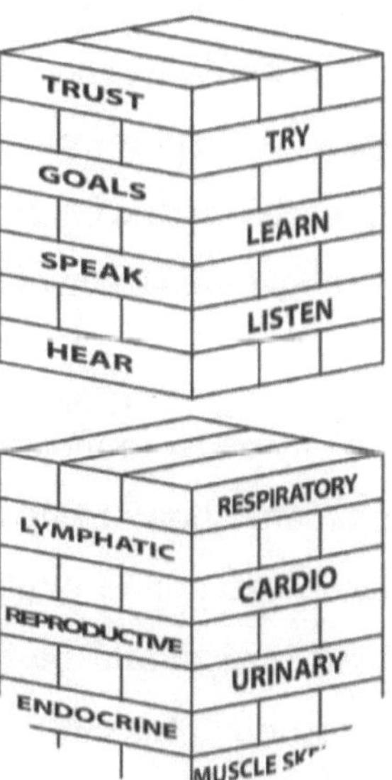

+ colossal communication

Trust and Respect; What Can I Do to Build a Strong Foundation?

It bears repeating: communication is key. Communication with yourself, connecting with your needs in a way that inspires trust and respect within yourself. This paves the path for finding the right people—people with compassion, trust, and respect for you and your ever-changing health needs. Your healthcare team members should adhere to these principles. This principle is inter-woven with the communication layer in your matrix.

You have the right to feel heard.

You are responsible for building and maintaining the foundation, or the principles for your own health. This includes collecting a strong, trusted healthcare team. This is very important. We have been laying down the foundation by reconnecting with your body's signals. With who you are and what your needs are in each moment. From a place of self-love, you now use trust, respect, compassion, non-judging and positive attitude to make decisions and communicate. And from these qualities will grow a strong foundation of team-work within your chosen healthcare team.

A structure is only as strong as its foundation. If you build a house over a sink pit, it doesn't matter how strong the walls are, your house will still sink. Once that foundation is built, finding and building a team to support your self-care should be easier, because you now know what qualities are important to you.

You have built the Selfcare Matrix on a foundation of the core values of Change. Integrated within that matrix are systems that make up

YOU and your key communication skills. A matrix consists of moving parts, so what is easy today might not be so easy tomorrow. Remain flexible with yourself and your expectations. You now have a matrix from which to build your team and selfcare goals.

> *"Don't Think Outside the Box. Think Like There is No Box."*
>
> — *Motivation Project*

Your team support should come from all areas of your life, not just the medical world. You are looking for guides, not dictators. Your friends, family, and the medical professionals that you trust and respect should all be part of your healthcare team. They each serve different roles but will help guide you along your selfcare journey. Each person on your team should be a partner in your selfcare needs.

A partner supports and guides you toward whatever your goals are from day to day, moment to moment. Let's break down your healthcare partners into two teams: friends and family become your "circle of trust," and medical professionals become your "dream team."

Try This: What Does a Partner Mean to Me?

Now, based on the exercises done earlier in the book, answer the following questions (there are no right or wrong answers):

- ***What is important to you in a partner?***
- ***Do you want to do all the talking, while they just listen?***
- ***How active are they in helping you set goals?***
- ***Do you want them with you every step of the way, or just when you ask?***

- *Do they need to anticipate your every move?*
- *Do they need to make your appointments, or drive you to the gym?*
- *Do you want them to tell you which practitioners to see?*
- *Do you want them to give you several suggestions so that you can decide what's best for you?*

How Do I Define My Healthcare Team?

Whole body health should include all medical professionals. In Chapter 3, I established the six systems that contribute to your health and wellness, that make one whole you. To address whole body health, your healthcare team needs to positively contribute to all the systems: Biological, Physical, Social, Emotional, Spiritual, and Mental. You define what is healthy for you in each category and how people, situations, work, and your community contribute to these systems. Your decisions will now be based on your awareness of what your current needs are.

Let's revisit your answers from the Chapter 4, exercise #3. Feel free to do the exercise again.

Try This (Again): Interpret What You Hear

Continue to be aware of your slow breathing. Now, you are going to explore your comfort level in each of your six systems. There are no right or wrong answers; just check-in and hear. Pretend you are a detective searching for signals that apply to each of your systems. You are looking for a comfort level score.

On a scale of 0 to 10, how comfortable are you in each of the following areas. Zero equals complete and total comfort, happiness, a sense of relaxation, and no pain or discomfort noted. Ten is extreme discomfort. This area is screaming at you for attention.

- *Biological (B): After breathing three or four times, things may be more quiet or calm within your environment. What is your state of health? Do you feel stuck? Do you fail to see improvement in your health no matter what you do? The first thought or answer is all you need. Hear it, then move on to the next system. It does not matter if you agree.*
  Score 0 1 2 3 4 5 6 7 8 9 10.

- *Physical (P): After breathing three or four times, go to the first area you feel in your body. (For example, "Right now, I get drawn to my right butt cheek as I'm sitting on this chair.")*
  Score 0 1 2 3 4 5 6 7 8 9 10

- *Mental (M): Are you able to focus on the breathing, or are you distracted? Does stopping to breathe and "checking in" feel impossible, or do you hate these types of exercises? No judgment, just listen. Where do you feel it in your body? What do you feel?*
  Score 0 1 2 3 4 5 6 7 8 9 10

- *Emotional (E): This is typically heard or felt in the abdomen and/or heart region. What's the first feeling that comes to mind? No right or wrong, only objective observation; no personal opinions. This is self-awareness.*
  Score 0 1 2 3 4 5 6 7 8 9 10

- *Social (S): When you think of your relationships with others, how does it feel in your body? Where do you feel it in your body? Do you feel more tense, more relaxed, happy, or sad?*
  Score 0 1 2 3 4 5 6 7 8 9 10

- *Spiritual (SP): What feeling does this word or topic evoke in your body? Do you feel that you have a purpose on this earth? Do you have a sense of connection and support? How strong is your will and determination to improve your health and achieve your goals? Where do you feel it in your body? What do you feel?*

  Score 0 1 2 3 4 5 6 7 8 9 10

Depending on when you are reading this, your scores have very likely changed from the last time that you answered them. Common sense would tell you that maybe you should focus on the system that currently has the highest score. Which healthcare team member could guide you towards improved health in this area? Remember, you are also a member of this team, and nothing in this world is truly separate.

You cannot separate your emotional health from your physical health. If you feel physically unhealthy, then you're not going to choose to go out. Now your social health is affected. You isolate yourself, and your mental and spiritual health can easily decline. Just as your body is a part of your whole health, so too should be your healthcare team. You need people on your team who support and guide you toward health in all systems.

An integrative approach should not be considered alternative or complimentary—not separate from your primary health care team. An integrative approach, equal participation, is the only supportive structure strong enough from which to build upon your foundation of self-care.

What are My First Priorities?

Let's explore all the potential healthcare team members for your team. Then re-prioritize them based on improved awareness of your selfcare needs. Hopefully, you have now become more aware of how your mental and emotional health affects your physical health. And that your biological health represents the best foundation upon which your health must be built.

As discussed in chapter 5, the basics of survival—being able to move, eat and drink, pee and poop, have sex, or make babies, and interact or connect with others—need to be present to function in this life. When these basic needs are disrupted, our purpose and quality of life can fall apart. A good example of this is cancer. Cancer cells attack you from the inside and can slowly break down your internal systems one-by-one, affecting your heart, lungs, brain, muscles, and so on. You can become dependent on others to dress and feed you or machines to breathe for you. Losing your independence can negatively affect your mood, your social and spiritual health. Depending on many factors, this decline can happen very slowly or it can happen rapidly.

So, our priorities should always start with your biological health. Since your biological and physical health can break down the other systems, your priorities in selfcare should start here. You need to be on board and on time with annual physical exams with your general doctor. Stay on schedule for your breast exams (mammograms), gut and rectal health (colonoscopies), and sex organ health (urologists, gynecologists). And don't forget your pregnant body and your growing baby's health (obstetrician). This will help decrease the need for emergency visits, only going to the doctor when you are sick or in emergent need. Having conversations when you are generally well frees up time to focus on your selfcare goals for the future. You can now use your dream team to guide you toward meeting your health and wellness goals for the future. This will help decrease the need for emergency reactive solutions and immediate relief reactions such as injections, medication and surgery.

What Leads My Need for Care?

First and foremost, if selfcare is the foundation of your healthcare, then mindfulness or self-awareness leads your need for care. If you are to put selfcare as the foundation of healthcare, then we need to change the priority structure of your healthcare team and how you use them. You now seek and use medical professionals in a proactive manner. Your decisions to seek care should be based on certain factors: Is your quality of life slowly being affected by pain and discomfort? If your answer is YES, act now. DO NOT WAIT until your quality of life is severely altered by pain, illness, or dysfunction. Most often, we can stop the latter by acting as soon as we have awareness of the former.

If you discuss the minor anxiety, aches, or pains at your wellness visits, then proactive solutions are more likely to work well for you. If more of us start to think and act in this way, then we will begin to re-arrange how everyone looks at our healthcare team priorities. I propose that we re-organize how and when we seek care.

Currently, most us only seek healthcare when our quality of life is very altered by pain or disability. We need immediate relief and are desperate enough to try anything. Medication, injections and surgery are necessary and effective, but should not be your first line of action. There can be severe side effects to all three.

Your first line of action should be paying mindful attention to your whole body every day. And that does not mean altering your life, but rather paying attention, knowing that there are reasons for every sensation. Ask many people why they have back pain, and often they will say, "It's because I am not as active as I should be," or my favorite, "Because I am old." Most often, you know the reason for your pain. You know why you are not able to do the things that you used to do; things that made you happy and gave you joy and purpose. Sorry, but age is not an excuse.

Making the decision to put your selfcare first every day, means changing the way you seek and use healthcare. There is a time and a place to use every discipline in the medical field.

Avoiding the need for emergent use
of your team should be your priority.

I know what you are thinking... "I am super healthy and do not need a doctor, let alone a team. I do everything I can to avoid needing them." That is awesome, but there will come a time where you need one. Whether it is an accident, appendicitis, or some emergency that causes you to end up in the ER, you will need healthcare. It is matter of "when," not "if." And after you leave the hospital, you will need to follow up with a doctor to help guide you toward the next steps. Wouldn't you rather have one you already know and trust? And, believe me, you would rather have one set up before the need arises.

How Do I Manage my Own Healthcare?

I propose that we break down our healthcare teams into three categories. For support and maintenance of your selfcare matrix use the "Selfcare Support" team. The "Life Support" team is there to help you stay on top of biological health. Being proactive with this team should take priority over emergency use. However, emergencies will happen in life and that's when we need our "Emergency Support" Team.

Yes, I am turning things around here. Just like making up words, I am proposing that we change our priorities and therefore the order of how we prioritize, and use, our teams. And, yes, I am therapy-biased, but therapy is a natural, conservative approach to healthcare. It aims to avoid drugs and surgery, avoiding the need for emergent use of your team. Therapy's very reason for existing is to educate you on how to care for yourself through hands-on approaches, as well as how to observe and analyze the causes with the result of independent, long-term solutions. You are hearing more and more in the media that we are over-dependent on medications, particularly pain drugs such as addictive narcotics. Therapy is the solution for avoiding those types of medications.

If you are hearing pain or dysfunction in your body, seek physical or occupational therapy before you turn to medications, injections and surgery. If you have already tried medications and surgery, therapy is still necessary to retrain the systems and bring normal function back into your life. If medication and surgery are still needed, your mind and body are better prepared and can improve your outcomes. Your dream team should combine effective, respectful communication between you, your selfcare support team, and your life support team. Remember, you are the most important member of each team. In fact, you are the leader and your circle of trust is there to support and guide you along the way.

What Does My Self-Healthcare Team Look Like?

Have you ever seen the picture of the iceberg sitting above water? The caption of the picture is "Success" and it shows that with successful people or situations you only see the little iceberg poking out of the water. What you don't see is the rest of the iceberg, which is huge, below the waters' surface. Your Self-Healthcare Team model follows this concept. Your selfcare is the foundation of the model, what everything else rests on or is built from. The majority of the hard work is done by you. You then utilize your all of the members of your team throughout your journey as needed.

My Self-Healthcare Team

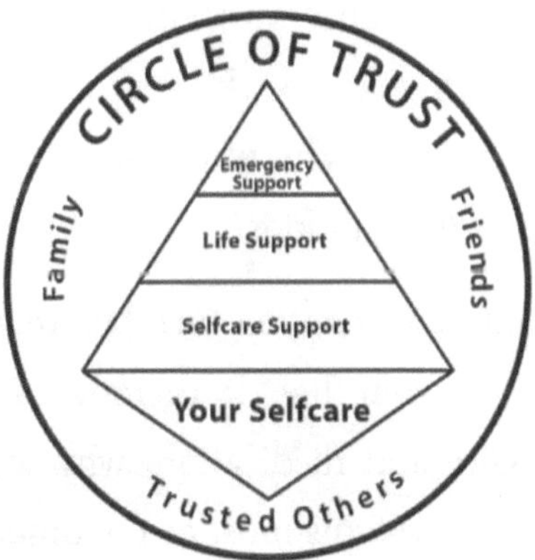

1. Selfcare Support Team—Now that we understand the importance of being mindful of our bodies' daily signals, our number one self-care priorities should revolve around supporting and maintaining the most important survival functions of the human body. As we learned in chapter four; moving, breathing, eating, peeing and pooping, balanced hormones, and having sex to keep up the species. Disciplines that are experts in these fields are:

A. You—Remember, no one knows your body as well as you do. You are the board member, the leader of each and every team.

B. Physical and Occupational Therapy (neuromuscular and musculoskeletal experts)—The focus of therapy is to guide you towards re-learning how to function in day-to-day life while avoiding medication and surgery or complementing them as needed. This group is not best used only when you can no longer function optimally. They are experts in how you should move and function optimally. They analyze or study how your body has learned to adapt in ways that are no longer working for you, hence the signals. Therapists will help you understand the "bad" habits and teach you good habits to build upon for the rest of your life. The education alone, because we spend one-on-one time with you, is worth its weight in gold. So why wait until you have more bad habits than good habits? Why wait until pain is so bad that you can't work or play with your kids?

This group should be where you turn before an emergency has a negative impact on your life. If therapy can help improve or complement surgery and medication, why would you not try it first? Insurance supports this most of the time. And if it does not, remember that your body is all you get in this life. Investing in your life should be your highest priority. Most clinics offer free screenings or consultations to meet and interview therapists and decide if therapy is right for you.

The power of touch is also essential for personalized care. Your therapists and your medical team should lay their hands on you. Assessing your tissue health and joint movement is extremely important at most of your health care appointments.

C. Integrative Medical Physicians—These experts will look at your entire medical history and help you coordinate your current medical team and look at you as a whole-body rather than only on a biological or physical level. They will ask questions to help you understand the current health of all six of your "bodies" that make you, you. Most hospital systems employ these types of physicians. Insurance most often covers these services.

D. Structural Support Team—There is no specific order; instead it is up to you to find what/who helps you achieve your goals.

    i.   Chiropractors
   ii.   Massage therapists
  iii.   Naturopaths
  iv.   Napropaths
   v.   Other body workers: Craniosacral therapists, reiki

E. Mental/Emotional Support—

- Psychiatry/psychology: If not a specific person, then someone with whom you can discuss mental and emotional health.
- Small circle of trusted friends and family who meet your needs based on the previous "partner question."

F. Movement Support Specialists—If you don't move, you are dependent on others to do everything for you, or face death—which many of us would rather do than relying on others to wipe our butts. Once you have been given an individualized plan by your OT or PT regarding your current movement needs, you need to commit to it daily. It does not stop when you walk out of the door. Not everyone feels comfortable in gyms, whether they are promised non-judgment or not. Finding what brings you joy is what matters here. Dancing in your bedroom works well but having guides to support you is what helps keep you motivated and accountable.

- Personal trainers
- Athletic trainers
- Gyms
- Yoga studios
- Pilates
- Group interactions where individualized movement and self-awareness are encouraged and supported (martial arts, water classes, etc...)

G. Social and Spiritual Support—

- A small circle of trusted friends and family who meet your needs based on the previous partner questionnaire.
- Religious or spiritual leaders and a community who support your beliefs, goals, and self-care needs.
- Support groups (live people are preferred, but here is a place for social media interactions that are controlled and only leave you feeling positive, happy, and supported).

2. Life Support Team—As described earlier, this team supports your basic life needs in a way that promotes you taking action before it is either an emergency or too late to achieve the results you really want. Supporting the best biological and physical health for a lifetime of wellness that supports—not defines—your quality of life. This is not about utilizing this team only when there are emergencies, but rather as your primary guides in this life: Biological and Physical Health Support.

A. You—Reporting your needs based on your awareness on a yearly and as-needed basis.

B. Primary Care Team—Supports cell health (experts in how all the systems interact on a basic level) and can guide you through the maze of options, which include medication and surgery, but with the primary goal of inspiring independent self-care rather than dependence on medication and surgery.

- General doctor—also known as primary care physician or internal medicine doctor.
- OBGYN— supports your pregnant body and the new life and growth of your baby:
  o Pregnancy Support
  o Midwife
  o Doula
  o Pediatrician

C. Secondary Care Team—Based on the guidance of your trusted primary care team and based on your clinical needs, concerns and test results. There is no certain order here, it will depend on your health needs.

- Other Therapy:
  - Speech
  - Respiratory
- Orthopedic (joint and movement health)
- Spinal (spinal, joint and movement health)
- Urology (urinary system health)
- Gynecology (sexual and hormone health)
- GI (pooping system health)
- Rheumatology (joint health)
- Endocrinologist (gland and hormone health)
- Neurologist (brain health)
- Podiatrist (foot and ankle joint health)
- Audiologist (ear and hearing health)
- Ear, nose, throat (hearing, breathing, swallowing health)
- Pain Management (emergency pain relief)

3. Emergency Support Team—

- Surgical Team
- Oncology (cancer)
- Emergency room doctors, nurses, radiologists, etc…

What Are My Team Priorities?

Understand that your team priorities will change based on your current state of health. And I am sure that I missed categories and professions that I have yet to encounter on my own journey. None of them is less important than the other when the need arises. Urology will move to the forefront if you're having issues with peeing. Knowing you have options is key, but only if you speak up. All your team members are there to GUIDE you.

You have the right and responsibility to yourself to make the final decision. This is based on the guidance of your team and intelligent, rational decision-making with the help of your circle of trust. But know that you are the one who must live with your decisions.

Review your patient's rights and responsibilities when choosing and interacting with your team members. Only you can determine whether they are right for you. If not, keep looking, asking, searching, and researching. Don't settle; keep looking.

After using and discussing the questions from Chapter 5 with your potential healthcare team member, answer this checklist of questions to help you determine whether they are right for you. Discuss your answers with those in your "circle of trust."

Your Dream Team = Your Circle of Trust + Your Ideal Health Care Team

Try This: **Are They Right for Me?**

1. Do I feel heard and supported?
2. Did they clearly define why, how, what I need to do to meet my goals in a way that I can understand?
3. Do I have a clear plan for what I need to do next?
4. What is my gut feeling during and after meeting with this person?
5. Did they take the time to listen?
6. Did I communicate my needs clearly? Was their advice based on my clear communication of my needs and goals?

How Do I Find Them?

Whom do you trust for simple everyday questions? Where do you look for the answers to your daily needs whether it's food, hair care, or childcare?

You need to have a circle of trust when it comes to who and where to find answers to our burning questions in every aspect of our life. You trust people you know first and foremost—certain friends and family members. Then you trust the people who are trusted by the people you trust—your friends' friends and maybe their family. Then you turn to other people in your circle, such as coworkers, your children's friends and families, their teachers, your teachers, or healthcare administrators. And when it comes to online information, you read reviews, look for balanced reviews. Know that many people only write a review out of anger or stress, which doesn't necessarily reflect the truth about that business or profession and their practice as a whole. If there are twenty-four 5 star reviews and only one or two fewer than three-star reviews, then that provider deserves a chance. Remember:

- Trust your gut.
- Don't believe everything you read or hear.
- Hear and feel for yourself.
- Don't give up.
- Once you find the right provider for your healthcare team and that person passes the "Are You Right for Me?" questions, they become part of your dream team and that resource can now be part of your circle of trust.
- Write a five-star review to help others find and create their circle of trust.

What is Important to Me?

We often tend to respond to comments such as "nice staff" or "comfortable waiting room." While those things are important what you are looking for are life changes. The reviews you are looking for should include comments from people whose lives have been changed. Comments such as "I can run without pain again," I can travel with my family for the first time in years," or "my doctor saved my life by listening to me and ordering the right tests." Go into your search with the specifics of what you are looking for in mind. Where are you now, where do you want to be, what type of guidance do you need, what needs to be improved so that your quality of life is what you want. Then, look for people making comments that relate to your needs.

Once you find the right provider for your healthcare team
and that person passes the "Are You Right for Me?" questions,
they become part of your dream team. Those resource can now be
part of your circle of trust.

Keep an Open Mind, Find and Open Mind?

Many of us are limited to the healthcare systems that our insurance allows. But there are usually many options within that system or systems. And often doctors' caseloads are full, and you cannot get on their patient list. However, if your close friend or family member is currently seeing one of those doctors, and they highly recommend them for you, they might be able to ask if the doctor is willing to take on another patient. Or ask to go on their waitlist.

If not, many systems are hiring nurse practitioners to help doctors out. Do not discount nurse practitioners as a major player on your team. They are typically easier to get in to see, and therefore can often spend more time with you. I have yet to meet one that does not exude compassion. The compassionate medical practitioner understands the importance of connection. And as you may have found in life, like-minded people tend to have good connections with people who share their philosophies and passions.

Health care professionals understand the power of compassion and truly connecting with their patients, read books or articles published by other professionals, attend conferences and classes about the subject, and seek other healthcare team members like themselves. They seek out others that will help support their patients. They realize that this is what truly helps them help their patients. And yes, once people find these wonderful healthcare professionals, it becomes hard to schedule with them, and they are often behind in their schedule.

Remember that they are worth the wait, so give them slack. The expectations and schedules for many health care professionals are becoming increasingly difficult to balance. They struggle, too. Finding the right team member for you is the goal, so enter the relationship with an open mind, and let them guide you, based on your questions and pre-set goals.

PRINCIPLE #8:

MAKE IT WORK FOR YOU

"Continuous improvement is better than delayed perfection."

— *Mark Twain*

Your Selfcare Matrix

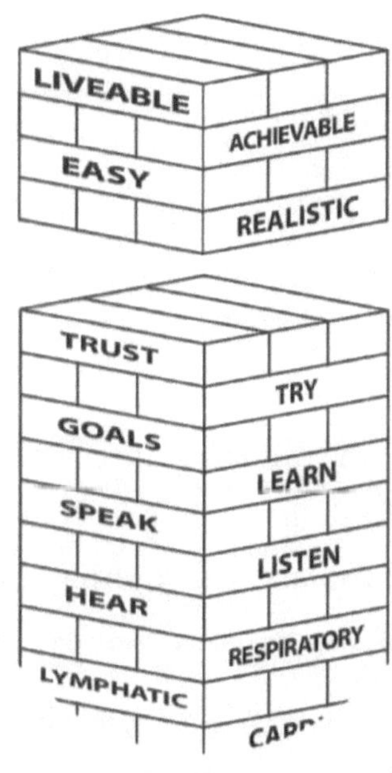

+ REAL goals

Flexible, Achievable Goals: Is That Even Possible?

What you expect of yourself— otherwise known as your goals— should be based on your core values now known as CHANGE. Your goals should not be so rigid that you will never meet them. Life is stressful and stress means change. In his book, *Full Catastrophe Living*, Jon Kabat-Zinn discusses life as a catastrophe. Most of us think of that word as a bad thing, a major disaster. But he states that it is really meant to show us the whole of our life experience, which is huge. Life is stressful, with constant ups and downs.

There is no permanence; there is only change. And not only do our bodies change, but so do our thoughts, opinions, jobs, relationships, possessions, friends, goals, everything.

So, our goals need to have room for change; again, we're not aiming for perfection.

Your Goals need to be REAL:

- ✓ REALISTIC
- ✓ EASY
- ✓ ACHIEVABLE
- ✓ LIVEABLE

Going into this with the thinking that you have total control is another way to set yourself up for failure. Your body and its needs are always changing, so if you are truly hearing, listening, and speaking, your goals will easily fit into the ebb and flow of each of your days.

There is no right or wrong way to set goals for yourself. Setting goals that you can actually meet is the only thing that matters. If you set the bar too high, then it is too easy to give up. Let's break up your goals into achievable timelines and categories. Your goals should support the six systems that make you YOU. Being aware of how your goals address each of your systems' needs will help you balance those needs as they change.

I know I am guilty of only addressing my biological and physical needs and therefore, I am just surviving day by day, rather than thriving. I often neglect my social and spiritual needs simply because I am too busy. I need daily reminders, because the more make time to pray, meditate, or spend time with friends, the more motivated I am to keep doing it. I feel good afterwards, every time. I feel empowered, healthy, and more energized to do the things I want to do that I enjoy and that make me happy. I see it work with my patients. It has helped me survive through chronic illness, one day at a time, which is really all that matters.

What are my REAL Goal Guidelines?

The foundation for setting goals is the Self-care Matrix and its core values of CHANGE. Your guideline for setting goals, something you can be successful at, is REAL. Your goals need to be **realistic, easy** to **achieve**, and ones you can **live** with every day. Livable means the goal helps make life worth living, adding to your joy. So not only living with your goal, or self-expectation, today, but every day. Will it move and grove with you in every moment of your life? Drinking six to eight ounces of water every day is a good goal but not if you're flying and traveling all day. Here is how to apply the guidelines of REAL goal-setting within the foundation of your core values of CHANGE.

*Is it something that makes you **consistently** feel **healthy** based on self-**awareness** whenever you check in here and **now**, moment by*

*moment? Will it help you **grow** forward?*
*Does it leave you feeling grateful and **empowered**?*

1. Is it **realistic** and **easy**? Can you be consistent with it every day? If not, can you forgive yourself and move on and do it when you remember? Don't let failure in this moment be an excuse to not do self-care the next moment/day/or month.
2. Does it make you feel healthy? Happy/better than when you started/hopeful?
3. Can you really **achieve** it every day? Does it allow you to feel aware? In your body? How you feel with others?
4. Does it remind you to be here, now, in the moment and out of your head if only one time each day?
5. Does it improve your life? Make you happy? Is it **livable**, comfortable? Does it allow or encourage you to grow? If not, can you let go and try something else? Ask for help on how to do that? Whether or not you achieve the goal today, can you be grateful for the opportunity to try, every day?
6. Does it help you feel empowered in your own health and wellness journey? Or do you feel that others are in control? Do you feel heard when you speak up about your goals?

What Do Healthy Habits Look Like for Me Throughout My Day?

Your goals need to cover every aspect of your life. I broke it down into the three categories listed below. Even if you do not currently work, professional goals could apply to your volunteer time or whatever occupies your time outside of your personal circle. If it does not apply, then simply set goals for personal and healthcare team categories.

1. Quickly answer the following questions. Go with the first answer to pop into your head. Do not spend any amount of time thinking – I'm looking for your gut instinct. Try to answer with three words or less, such as good, fair or poor.

2. What is your current state of health in each of the six systems? Biological Physical Mental Emotional Social Spiritual

3. What was it before?

4. How has it changed?

5. What do you want it to be? (Your "ideal" state of health)

6. What are you willing to do to achieve it?

7. How can you stay positive in your mindset if you are unable to achieve your "ideal" state of health?

Now take those answers and break them into very broad statements regarding what you would like to change regarding your whole-body health.

Try This: **Happy, Healthy, Whole You**

1. Spend five minutes just writing down what whole-body health looks like on you this year. Write like crazy, don't think, just write whatever comes to you. Include what you would like to do more of. Where would you do it? Who would you do it with? What would it take to get you there? Who do you have that can help? Who do you need to help get you there?

2. Next, circle the most realistic, easy, achievable, and livable aspects of what healthy looks like for you.

3. Then think about what aspects of your life you could apply these goals to. Break that down into three categories:

   a. Personal

b. Professional

c. Healthcare team

Here are some examples:

- I want to feel less stressed at work.
- I want more energy so that I can…(play with my kids at the end of the day or cook more and eat out less).
- I want to lose 10 pounds.
- I don't want my social life controlled by my fibromyalgia/chronic pain.
- I want to have less back pain.
- I want to not leak urine when I laugh with my friends.
- I want to make friends this year.
- I want to find a community of people that share my spiritual beliefs.
- I want to eat healthier.
- I want guidance with my physical exercise routine.
- I want guidance with my daily self-care routine.
- I want to find a doctor who shares my values.

Refer to your answers and break them down as they fit into each category listed below and consider "reasonable" and "achievable" timelines. Is it possible or necessary to achieve them today or this week? Remember, setting yourself up for success is what matters the most. Using the CHANGE core values and REAL goal-setting guidelines and applying them toward the Whole You: 6 Systems is your key to success. It is how you will achieve your whole-body health potential.

Categories:

1. Personal
   a. Biological: Consistent Healthy Awareness Now Grow Empowerment
   b. Physical: Consistent Healthy Awareness Now Grow Empowerment
   c. Spiritual: Consistent Healthy Awareness Now Grow Empowerment
   d. Emotional: Consistent Healthy Awareness Now Grow Empowerment
   e. Mental: Consistent Healthy Awareness Now Grow Empowerment

2. Professional
   a. Biological: Consistent Healthy Awareness Now Grow Empowerment
   b. Physical: Consistent Healthy Awareness Now Grow Empowerment
   c. Spiritual: Consistent Healthy Awareness Now Grow Empowerment
   d. Emotional: Consistent Healthy Awareness Now Grow Empowerment
   e. Mental: Consistent Healthy Awareness Now Grow Empowerment

3. Healthcare Team
   a. Biological: Consistent Healthy Awareness Now Grow Empowerment
   b. Physical: Consistent Healthy Awareness Now Grow Empowerment

    c. **Spiritual: Consistent Healthy Awareness Now Grow Empowerment**

    d. **Emotional: Consistent Healthy Awareness Now Grow Empowerment**

    e. **Mental: Consistent Healthy Awareness Now Grow Empowerment**

Timelines:

1. **Today**
2. **This week**
3. **This month**
4. **This year**

What Are My REAL Personal Goals?

Continue to use your previous answers and set personal goals. Which system needs the most attention at this moment? This will help you determine where to begin. When you stop, breathe and check in, what are you hearing? What do you find you need in this moment as you listen and investigate further? Starting with a personal goal will be the easiest, as your body will tell you what your most immediate need is, such as hunger or discomfort. So, start with the personal category and a timeline.

Now that you understand that whole-body health refers to balanced health of all six systems, you can see how each goal can—and should—positively affect them. This allows your goals to contribute to your health and wellness in a balanced way.

Applying the Selfcare Matrix with the core values of CHANGE
will help ensure that your goals are about independent selfcare
and not about pleasing others or setting unrealistic goals.

Examples include:

My **personal** goal for **today** (It can change every day, or you can make it "today" and "this week"—it's whatever you want. You got this!)

- When I wake up I will __________ [smile to myself / smile at a stranger / say "Thank you, God, it's great to be alive!] (mental, emotional, social, spiritual)
- Walk for 10 minutes. (physical)
- Drink three bottles of water. (biological, physical)
- Do one thing that makes me happy. (mental, emotional, social, spiritual)
- Hear and listen to what my body needs. (all six)
- Stretch my hips, go for a walk, etc... (physical)
- Spend time with my pet. (mental, emotional, physical)
- Spend five minutes just sitting and breathing or praying.
- Read one chapter of a book to help me grow. (mental, emotional, spiritual)

My **personal** goal for this **week**:

- Walk (or exercise of choice) three times for 10 minutes this week. (physical)
- Eat my favorite food one time this week. (mental, emotional)
- Eat food that makes me feel good, happy, energetic at least three times this week. (biological, physical)
- Meet a friend or friends for coffee. (mental, emotional, social)

- Write in my journal three times. (mental, emotional, social)
- Be intimate with my partner.
- Read a book about your spiritual beliefs. (mental, emotional, social, spiritual)
- Just sitting and breathing and/or praying for 10 minutes three to five times this week. (biological, mental, emotional, spiritual)
- We will eat together at the dinner table at least one time a week. (social, mental, emotional)

My **personal** goal for this **month**:

- Increase my water intake to five bottles of water per day. (biological, physical)
- Walk, move, exercise in ways that make me happy and feel good five times a week for at least three weeks. (biological, physical, mental, emotional)
- Stretch 10 minutes a day at least three times a week for the next four weeks. (biological, physical, mental, emotional)
- Sit and be quiet at least one day per week this month. (spiritual, mental, emotional)
- Try three "new" healthy foods or recipes each week this month. (biological, physical)
- Read a book purely for entertainment at least one time this month. (social, mental, emotional)
- Read a book or articles about health-related topics least one time this month. (biological, physical, mental, emotional)
- Try just sitting and breathing and/or praying for five minutes 10 times this week. (biological, mental, emotional, spiritual)
- Set a monthly date night with partner or coffee time or phone time with friends. (social)

My **personal** goal for this **year**:

- Go visit one new place.
- Learn a new…. (instrument, sport, game, hobby, occupation).
- Connect with my partner on a deeper level.
- Figure out what makes me happy through experimenting this year.
- I will take a class in something that I have wanted to learn for fun. (mental, emotional)
- Develop a routine for simply being, whether it is breathing/meditating, praying, going to church, or whatever that means to you.

What Are My REAL Professional Goals?

Can I tell you a big secret? Not everyone loves his or her job. Many people hate their jobs or feel stuck in a rut, which leaves you with two choices. And yes, they are your choices. You can choose to blame life or others for the job you are in, but you get to choose what you do about it. Either change the situation you're in—talk to your boss, ask for a promotion or change in hours or shifts, or apply for another job...OR change your attitude about the situation.

"Yes, I hate my job, but I have great benefits and will be able to retire comfortably..." or "It's close to home, it pays the bills, and feeds my family."

Choose to be positive as you go about your daily tasks and how you think and talk about your job and co-workers and your state of health will quite possibly change for the better too.

Choose to be positive about your work. Everyday.

Examples of professional goals:

My **professional** goals for **today** (this can change every day, or you can make it "today" AND "this week":

- When I wake up, I will...[smile to myself / say, "This will be a great day" / leave my personal "stuff" at the door when I walk into work today / strive to not take anything personal today]. (mental, emotional, social, spiritual)
- Park further away so I have to walk further or take the stairs at least one time. (physical)
- Every time I see water on my desk, I will take a sip. (biological, physical)
- Do one thing that makes me happy. (mental, emotional, social, spiritual)
- Hear and listen to what my colleague needs. (all six)
- Express my needs immediately when I feel... [frustration or anger] in my body. (all six)
- Express my needs immediately when I feel... [happy, excited] in my body. (all six)
- Congratulate a coworker immediately when I notice they did something to support me or the job. (mental, emotional, social)
- Ask a job leader about something I have wanted to learn but have been too scared to try/fail. (mental, emotional, physical)
- I will not think, talk about, or do anything related to work for one hour during my off hours.

My **professional** goal for this **week**:

- Read five chapters of a book/magazine/article/blog about something that I have wanted to learn to improve my skills or help me learn new skills. (mental, emotional)
- Have lunch with a coworker that I normally do not talk to.
- Read a book or an article about how to improve my social skills or leadership skills. (mental, emotional, social, spiritual)
- Try just sitting and breathing for five minutes, three times this week before or after eating or during a break. (biological, mental, emotional, spiritual)
- Walk 10 minutes during my break three times this week. (biological, physical)
- Congratulate a coworker immediately when I notice they did something to support me or the job three times this week. (mental, emotional, social)
- I will not think, talk about, or do anything related to work for two days during my off hours. (mental, spiritual, emotional)

My **professional** goal for this **month**:

- Increase my water intake to five bottles of water per day for the month. (biological, physical)
- Walk, move, exercise in ways that make me happy and feel good five times a week for at least three weeks. (biological, physical, social, mental emotional)
- Stretch 10 minutes a day at least three times a week for the next four weeks. (biological, physical, mental, emotional)
- Try three "new" healthy foods or recipes each week this month. (biological, physical, mental, emotional)

- Read a book this month that will improve my skills. (mental, social, emotional, spiritual)
- Read a book, blog, or article about any health-related topic at least one time this month. (biological, physical, mental emotional)
- Try just sitting and breathing for five minutes 10 times this week. (biological, mental, emotional, spiritual)
- I will bring lunch three times each week, 12 times each month to eat out less often, stay at work to eat with other, save money and eat more healthily. (biological, physical, mental, social, emotional)
- I will smile at/greet at least one person a day whom I have not met or talked to much, regardless of whether they smile back. Giving to give. (social, mental, emotional)

My **professional** goal for this **year**:

- I will take a class in something that I have wanted to learn to, (improve my skills, or qualify me to apply for a promotion, another job…). (mental, emotional)
- I will positively reinforce three co-workers (or one coworker three times, depending on how big my workplace is) each month either verbally or in writing. This could be a smile, a "thank you," or a "great job at…" (social, mental, emotional, spiritual)
- I will arrive five minutes earlier than usual one day a week each month so that I can breathe and center before starting my day. (biological, mental, emotional, spiritual)
- I will have an established stretching routine that I will do during and after work at least three times a week every month.

- I will talk to my job leader about an idea I have had with a solid plan to make it happen and a "Plan B" for my mental health if shot down. (mental, emotional, social, spiritual)

- I will take five minutes during my lunch or break time to stretch in ways for body parts that my body is telling me I need. (biological, physical)

- I will have a plan for healthy eating and drinking balanced with permission to eat less healthily in order to participate in work events without guilt. (physical, biological, mental, emotional, social, spiritual)

- I will use all my earned PTO this year and spend time with my family or in a place that I feel peaceful and happy. (biological, physical, social, emotional, social, spiritual)

What Are My REAL Healthcare Team Goals?

Your goal priorities here are going to be very different based on your current state of health. If you are anything like me, when I was very healthy and active my healthcare team goal was "avoid needing a healthcare team." But we all need a good team because no matter your current state of health, you will need a good doctor at some point.

In my practice, I often hear "I hate doctors," or "I hate medicine," which saddens me, because physicians, medicine, and surgery are there for a reason and that reason is your health and extending your life expectancy. And you will need a good doctor at some point in your life; there is no way around it. Accidents and illness are a part of life. As I said before, catastrophe is a fantastic way to look at the whole of life. Ups and downs make up your life. Avoiding surgery, medications, and injections is a much more realistic goal than avoiding doctors.

Doesn't it make sense then to have the choice to hand-pick a doctor that you like, to guide and support you whenever you need help with the ups as well as manage the downs? And as far as the statements of "I hate my doctor(s) and meds," I will apply the same strategy as to "hating" your job. You have two choices: change the situation or change your attitude. Remember Principle #2: Be aware of what's holding you back. You have to let go of the excuses before you can move forward and achieve your goals.

Your goal here is to meet your needs based on intelligent, educated awareness. This means your goals need to help you respect your gut feeling, and allow you to feel heard, respected, and in control of your choices. This will affect the health of ALL your whole-body health systems. Prioritize your healthcare team goals based on your previous general goals.

Refer to the communication skills checklist in Chapter 7 to help focus your healthcare team goal-setting.

Let's look at some examples of goal-setting for creating your ideal healthcare team. Keep in mind which of the six systems you need addressed. By addressing one you are often addressing all of them, so they are not listed below as with the previous goal examples.

My **health care team** goals for **today**:

- I will research what my choices are for a _______ [Primary Care Physician, Physical or Occupational Therapist, Naturopath, Nutritionist].
- I will reach out to someone on my team and ask a question I have been wanting to ask. (For example, how much water is healthy for me to drink?)

- I will communicate with my healthcare team member in a way that is positive and allows me to express my needs.
- I will write a list of what I heard today in my body to discuss with my doctor at my next visit. (And keep it somewhere where I will remember to bring it with me next time.)
- I will write a pros and cons list of my current health care team and determine who is positively contributing/guiding me and who is not.
- I will complete a task given to me by my health care team member. (For example, three exercises given to me by my PT.

My **health care team** goal for this **week**:

- Read reviews about doctors I have heard about, or found in my daily research, and ask question or interact with others that have experience with these doctors.
- Research and reach out to new healthcare professionals that I found I needed based on my pros and cons list.
- I will research groups, workshops, and health fairs that positively contribute to my self-care goals. (For example, back pain workshop, support group, painting class, book club.)
- I will congratulate one of my healthcare team members by sending a "thank you" card or email (yes, I have done this) when I notice they did something to support and guide me.
- I will complete a task given to me by my health care team member. (For example, do my home exercise program, consistently take my probiotic as prescribed, search out a massage therapist as recommended by my doctor or naturopath, introduce one new food into my diet per my nutritionist.)

My **health care team** goal for this **month**:

- I will be consistent with my home exercise program and take notes of what makes me feel better, and what doesn't, and bring the list with me to my next appointment.
- I will participate in a group or workshop that positively contributes to my self-care goals. (For example, chat group or support group.)
- I will write a positive five-star review on Google, Yelp, their website, or their Facebook page about the health care team professionals that were top on my pros and cons list to help others find and utilize this positive resource.
- I will read a book, article, or watch a video about a health care topic that is at the top of my general goals list, and write a list of questions about it to discuss with someone in my circle of trust.
- I will keep a list of what I heard in my body throughout this month, to discuss with my healthcare professional at my next visit (and put it where I will remember to bring it with me next time).
- I will find resources that will help me achieve my goals.

My **health care team** goal for this **year**:

- I will coordinate a team of healthcare professionals who guide, support and contribute positively to my self-care goals.
- I will have a plan for eating and drinking healthily and in a balanced way, based on discussions I have had with my health care team throughout the year (and based on blood work, diagnostic testing, and what I hear in my body).

- I will practice my rights and responsibilities and communication skills when interacting with anyone on my team, remembering that compassion and respect are a two-way street.
- I will eliminate people from my team that I have found do not hear and listen to my needs, are not guiding me, or supporting my sound choices.
- I will admit that needing a team of healthcare professionals and a circle of trust is necessary for my health and not a sign of weakness, ever.
- I will respond to my body when it "speaks," avoiding emergent situations when necessary, but knowing the difference between when my health is in a state of emergency and having a plan for when it occurs.

PRINCIPLE #9:

STAY FLEXIBLE

"Stay committed to your decisions but stay flexible in your approach."

— *Tony Robbins*

Your Selfcare Matrix

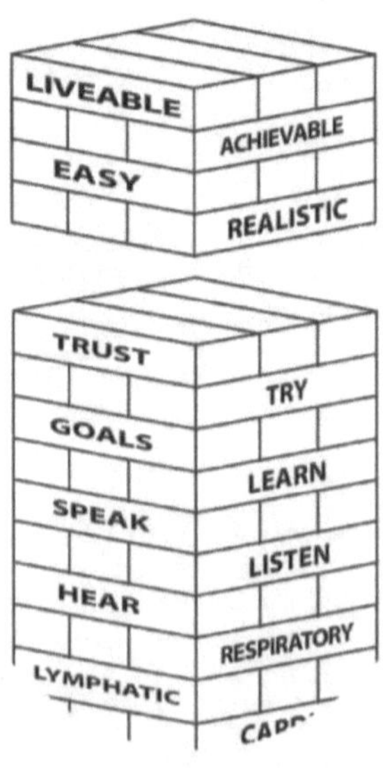

+ REAL goals

How Do I Make Lemonade out of My Situation?

"When life gives you lemons, make lemonade." We all know the saying, but have you ever noticed that it never says "IF" life gives you lemons? No. It always says "when" life gives you lemons. For the one constant in life is change. I can guarantee you that life will give you lemons; that change will happen. But the amazing gift is that you get to choose what to do with those lemons.

Truly identify with this phrase and you are on your way to taking back your healthcare. Adapting this phrase to your life is to be flexible. It changes how you think and behave, regardless of what life throws at you, whether it is illness, injury, sadness, death, tragedy—or even excitement and happiness.

Why Are Being Flexible and Adaptable Keys to My Success?

In occupational therapy our treatment goals are related to helping others become as independent as possible in any activity of daily living or "ADL." This includes dressing, toileting, peeing, pooping, showering, shopping with a friend or opening a jar. All these daily activities contribute to your "roles" in life. Your sense of purpose in this life and in the world. All any human wants in life really, is to have a purpose. The term "occupation" refers to any role in life, such as a mother, chef, a reader, a lover, a hiker, a computer engineer, or simply a human being. When pain, illness, or injury affect that independence, your purpose, happiness, health, and well-being are altered. To be successful in anything we learn to modify or adapt our environment, (also known as being flexible), so that we can still be independent, purposeful and happy.

You just had hip surgery and are not allowed to bend all the way to put on your shoes and socks. I teach you different ways to do it on your own. In the case of a child with cerebral palsy wanting to learn how to feed herself, I teach the child and the mother how to use special utensils, chairs and table heights. How to stretch or strengthen the muscles that she needs to use to have the best posture and get the spoon to her mouth.

In the case of a woman whose life is disrupted because she has a strong urge to pee 12 times a day and five times at night, I teach her how to modify or change her behaviors. Not drinking two pots of coffee or running to the bathroom every time she feels the faintest urge. Teach her how to gain control of her bladder and sleep restfully. Learning to breathe and control the panic associated with peeing her pants. Giving her an understanding of what muscles are involved so that she can gain control of them. Education is all part of how to become successful in selfcare while on her own personal journey.

Being flexible and adaptable is a huge key to success when it comes to anything that we want to achieve. We all want to be successful. That is what gives us confidence to do new things, to learn and grow. Not being flexible and adaptable can cause us to become stuck in a rut. If you don't try many ways to get your car out of a ditch—which may include asking for help from a tow-truck driver—then it will sit there and rust. It can no longer perform its intended purpose.

If I Don't Use It Will I Lose It?

When it comes to physical flexibility, I tell my patients that most of us get it free until about third grade, but after that, we must earn it every day, especially once we enter the workforce. Eventually, our lives become about performing the same motions repeatedly, whether you sit at a computer all day, or stand in a factory line. The same rule applies for exercise. If you only ever run, your muscles become used to the same few motions day in and day out. There must be balance in how you move. If we do not allow our muscles to move in all the different ways they were meant to move—shortening and lengthening, twisting, bending, reaching—then they become stuck in a rut too.

Stretching your muscles, moving in many ways, and being physically flexible are just as important as strengthening. Balanced physical health is about doing exercises that lengthen and strengthen the muscles. Running is very hard on the joints and is considered more of a "shortening, compressive" exercise for the body. Swimming is more of a lengthening, non-weight bearing exercise, so the two can balance one another out. I will challenge you in the next chapter with specific exercises to try.

Alternating days to swim and run—rather than only doing one or the other—is flexible thinking, which leads to balance. Equally important is spending a day hanging out with friends or family. Sitting in the sun reading, allowing for mental, emotional, social, and spiritual renewal, is a balanced approach to health. This is whole-body flexibility that we should strive to achieve.

I Need to Stretch My Mind Too?

Health is an integration of all systems; biological, physical, mental, emotional, and spiritual. It is balanced well-being. Flexibility must apply to all these systems as well. It is well known that there is research proving physical exercise is linked to overall improved health and wellness of our entire being, but did you know that there is also research proving that psychological flexibility is a fundamental aspect of health as well?

In the research article "Psychological Flexibility as a Fundamental Aspect of Health," it states, "...achieving psychological health is one of the foremost goals of human existence." *36* When looking at the three stories discussed earlier, it is easy to see how physical health and psychological flexibility are linked. If the man with the total hip replacement just gave up trying to put his socks on, he would instantly become dependent on his spouse to do this task for him for life. If he doesn't figure out how to adapt to the changes, or create new situations, his hip won't heal right, he'll have limited adventures with his wife and friends, and you get the point.

If the child never tries to learn to feed herself, despite her potential, she is dependent on others to feed her forever. This will affect her belief that she can learn anything new, and she will be a victim to the body into which she was born.

The woman who has a constant urge to pee due to poor bladder control lives in constant fear of leaving the bathroom or smelling like urine. She will isolate herself from friends and intimacy.

Giving up allows these people more time to sit and worry rather than participate in life. All three of these people's lives will be limited. They will pull away from society. Innately, we know that this will affect their quality of life and potential for happiness.

Why Does Having an Attitude of Gratitude Matter?

Psychological flexibility allows us to keep trying. Simply put, having a positive attitude, believing in yourself no matter what – that's what makes the difference between becoming stuck or achieving your goals. Using the positive focus on gratitude will steer you in the re-direction every time you fall off the track. Be thankful for what you do have right here, right now. This gives us the fuel to gather our mental, physical, and emotional willpower to keep fighting, to keep trying to find what works for us, every day. Add healthy spiritual beliefs and the fire keeps burning. Seeing the good in every lesson (which is what every failure and challenge truly is), and being thankful for it, that is a flexible mind. It gives you a sense of purpose; a belief that you are supported and never truly alone. Faith shows you that there is a higher purpose behind it all.

A lack of psychological flexibility means a closed mind. You will experience constant worry about the same things every day, believing that you have no control over anything. Nothing is your fault or responsibility. This type of belief system does not allow you to rebound from stressful or traumatic events. It makes it difficult to plan for or achieve goals. Once again, you become stuck in a rut with nowhere to go, nothing to do, no one to help you. Just a broken-down truck stuck in a hole with a bunch of lemons.

So, once you've set your goals and made plans to achieve them, expect your plan to change; allow for it. Your health will always change. Every day is a new opportunity to learn, listen, and change. If you expect it, you can control how you react to it and therefore get to choose what to do about it. That is mental and emotional flexibility. Your physical flexibility must be earned every day. Give your body's systems opportunities to explore different movements and re-learn new patterns. Be thankful for each and every signal lesson, failure and challenge. Adapt thinking patterns such as "if it hadn't been for this (e.g., Lyme disease), I never would have experienced that, (e.g., more time to be with my family and re-arrange my life priorities). Learning and growth is always something to be grateful for.

Try This: Grow and Let Go

1. *Take a moment to stop where you are and close your eyes. Take a couple of slow deep breaths and check in with how your body feels. The mind usually first goes to the place where there is tension or discomfort. These parts are talking to you. So, move them, stretch them as it feels good, and stop and check in again with the breathing. Keep your eyes closed. Notice a difference? Apply this throughout your day. Listen, learn, and act rather than react.*

2. *If you sit every day, try stretching in opposite positions; instead of bent knees and hips, try stretching the front of your hips and backs of your legs with straight knees*

3. *Identify what position you sit or stand in the most and change it up. Cross the other ankle, lean on the other arm rest, lunge with the other foot*

4. *Pay attention to your attitude in situations that you know upset you and those in which you struggle to maintain a good attitude. Be aware of how it feels in your body at the time. Try to stop and simply smile on the inside. Try something different. Notice the changes. Simply be aware, because that is how change begins. Don't judge. Just observe.*

PRINCIPLE #10:

FIND BALANCE

"The best and safest thing is to keep a balance in your life, acknowledge the great powers around us and in us. If you can do that, and live that way, you are really a wise man."

— Euripides

Your Selfcare Matrix

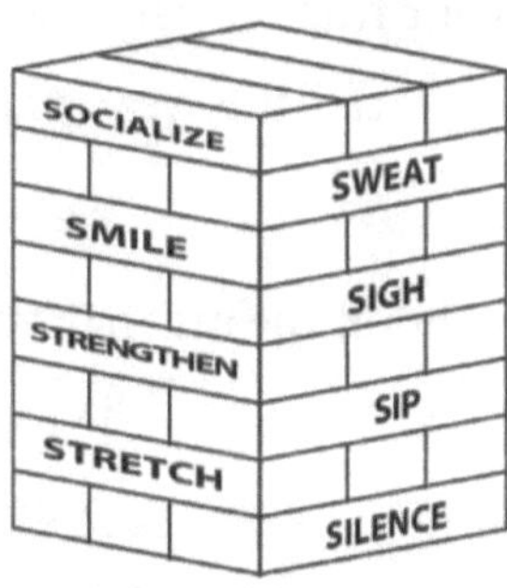

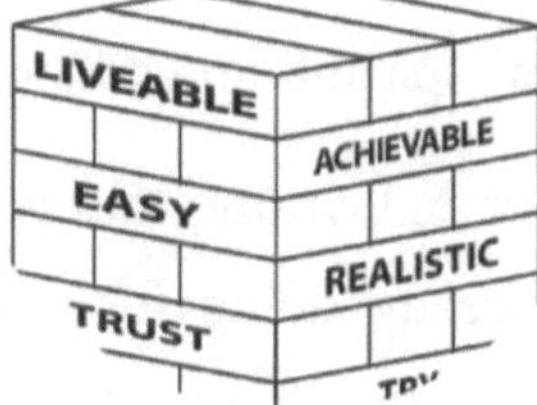

+ balanced living

What Does "Balanced Living" Mean for Me?

The goal of balance is not perfection. Balance is striving to pay attention to all your body's systems in a way that puts equal value on each system. Goal-setting in a balanced way allows you to see when one system receives less than its fair share of attention. This helps you better understand your needs, day by day, moment by moment. Ignoring your body's signals over the years can lead to illness and dysfunction. But listening day-to-day allows you to adapt your goals and habits to maintain balance.

If the signals continue and you know that you have tried to achieve your goals based on sound advice from your health care teams, you immediately know that it is time to ask for help. Hear, listen, and speak. Balancing your systems is about knowing when to trust your current knowledge of how your body works—within the realms of advice given to you by your trusted team—and when to seek further help. What keeps you balanced this year may change next year, or even next month.

Making it this far in the book means that you are committed. You now understand that to live a balanced life, you cannot look at your body and its needs as separate. Feeding your need for social contact and intimacy is not only for your social and mental health. It is also essential for your physical, spiritual and biological health.

And when thinking about and writing your goals, you saw how many great things you are already doing for yourself, because it ALL matters. Just sitting at the table with your family for dinner, enjoying a meal you prepared, attends to your social, mental, emotional, spiritual, physical, and biological health needs. See how easy that was?

How Does Balance Rely on My Self-Awareness?

All it takes is awareness. Seriously, that's it. This entire book just comes down to that. Be aware of what your body needs in this moment, today. From awareness comes improved communication, real goals, and a balanced life. Easy peasy.

In my day-to-day work with patients that live with long term/chronic dysfunction, we discuss balance during every session. But it is often very hard to see where in your life you're out of balance, because you've been doing it in the same way for years. When I approach therapy with my patients, I act as their guide. I call myself another person on their team. I explain how I will "hold a mirror" up to their day and help them see which habits are currently contributing to their health and which ones may not be. We all need this help at some point—if not many points—throughout our lives.

I once evaluated a woman for complaints of urinary urgency and frequency. She felt as though she was living in the bathroom or constantly seeking one out when in public, which was no fun at all. I always ask patients to fill out a "bladder diary" to show me their normal bladder habits. I teach about bladder irritants and how food and fluid can contribute to bowel, bladder, and pelvic floor problems. After I read the list of irritants, the woman's husband said that she had been eating the exact same way for years. They were curious as to how this could contribute to her current condition. I asked him to repeat that phrase "the exact same way for years."

Try This: Balanced Awareness

Your body's needs change, so your habits should change, too. Bring awareness to what you want to change. Be consistent. Make healthy choices. Hold a mirror up to your day, week, month, and year and ask yourself:

- *Am I living in balance, honoring all of my systems?*
- *Am I being consistent with my healthy choices through a place of awareness?*
- *Am I allowing my habits and goals to be real and in the moment?*
- *Am I grateful and able to let go?*
- *Am I being an empowered person? Asking for help, using my team?*

Answering "yes" to all of those questions is living within the Self-Care Matrix.

Hooray!

What are the 8 "S" Rules?

Now, let's explore some examples of how to live in balance using the Self-Care Matrix. Balancing your six systems and honoring your commitment to CHANGE is easy now that you have awareness. Remember your needs are different from every other person's and can change day-to-day. If you are ever unsure about what is right for you, what should you do? You can use the Matrix as your frame of reference. Then use your "circle of trust" and healthcare team accordingly.

Your "to do" list is simple.

- Drink water and eat in healthy moderation.
- Move.

- Breathe
- Smile.
- Be thankful.
- Forgive.

But we all know that the simple things are often the most difficult. Making selfcare your daily purpose in life is your power. Yes, even you're super power. This is your life. You get to choose—actually, you MUST choose. Happiness is a choice. I still struggle to this day with the after effects of Lyme disease. And this list is not always easy for me to check off every day. But I try, because I am committed. I do what I can everyday so that when I need my health care team, I am able to communicate my needs and frustrations so that I can receive the support and guidance I need. Do I judge myself when I fail at one of these things, such as drinking water? Why yes, yes, I do. But then I remember how grateful I am to be alive, and I forgive myself and move on.

And believe me, I get A LOT of practice forgiving myself. Keeping it simple is the only way for me to be successful, on both my good days and not-so-good days. The "to-do" list that tops the Selfcare Matrix is simple. It covers all the systems for your whole-body health; to live in balance. I know that you will be creative and eventually add more to each system. What I list below is a starting point. You get to choose where to go from there. Have fun and do what feels right for you. Most importantly, listen to your body.

1. Biological: Drink water and eat in healthy moderation. **SIP**
2. Physical: Move—balanced cardio, stretching, strengthening. **SWEAT, STRENGTHEN, STRETCH.**

3. Mental: Breathe and check in. **SIGH, SILENCE.**

4. Emotional: Breathe. Do one thing that makes you happy every day. **SIGH, SMILE**

5. Social: Connect, make eye contact, and smile to yourself and others. **SOCIALIZE**

6. Spiritual: Practice gratitude and forgiveness and determine your will today. **SILENCE, SMILE**

The 8 "S" Rules:

- **SIP**--refers to sipping water or tasting/eating healthy foods throughout the day, trying new things in small doses, and bringing new things into your life.

- **STRETCH** --Be flexible in all of your Six Systems, not just the physical.

- **STRENGTHEN** --not only your physical body, but also your convictions as well. Strengthen your spiritual self.

- **SWEAT** --refers to cardio health but also rejuvenation. It's about sloughing off the old to make room for the new.

- **SIGH**—take time to breathe for the sake of breathing and allow yourself to take time to just do nothing throughout the day. You only need a few moments to make a big difference.

- **SILENCE**— Take time to hear and listen, to connect to yourself and others.

- **SMILE**—Simply smile for no reason, to yourself and others.

- **SOCIALIZE**—Allow your world to grow from your inner circle to the outside world. Connect and reconnect. Learn, live, give love, get love.

Now let's put it all together into
Your Complete Selfcare Matrix

your selfcare matrix

Biological: How Does Drinking Water Every Day Keeps the Doctor Away?

As I have said, there is a time and a place to need a doctor in your life. But the goal for selfcare is to act and ensure that you need them on your terms—not as a very last resort or emergency option. Yes, the phrase use to be "an apple a day," but I have already established that I am rebelliously changing words, definitions, and now phrases.

SIP: Why, How Much and What?

Drinking water as your main source of fluid is one of the easiest ways to keep your biological system in balance. And remember, if your cells are not healthy—if they are wanting for anything—then every other system can easily fall out of balance. In his book, *Your Body's Many Cries for Water; You're Not Sick You're Thirsty*, Dr. F. Batmanghelidj tells his story of when he was imprisoned in another country and was asked to treat the other inmates.

He found that he was able to help almost every patient's symptoms by giving them water. He describes it as "basic economics." If you are not replacing the water in your body, then your body will take it from somewhere else—your blood, organs, and so on—and that can lead to many other problems that are way more difficult to heal. Now that you understand how we cannot separate selfcare from healthcare, the 6 systems from each other or the 11 systems that make up the body, check out these statistics.

Water is the basis of all life and that includes your body. Your muscles that move your body are 75% water; your blood, which transports nutrients, is 82% water; your lungs— that provide your oxygen—are

90% water; your brain, that is the control center of your body, is 76% water; even your bones are 25% water.[37]

Drinking a balanced intake of water has been shown to reduce headaches, constipation, kidney stones, improve weight loss, and even cure hangovers.[38]

I see this truth every day in my clinic. Every patient that we see receives "the water talk," whether they have bowel problems such as constipation, or bladder issues such as leakage, or difficulty peeing. Even people with chronic pain hear the lecture. And almost every patient who tracks his or her water intake over a three-day period is amazed to find that they do not drink as much as they thought. If you were to research how much water to drink, you would get many different answers. It really does vary per person.

SIP also refers to eating in healthy moderation throughout the day. If you are eating water-based foods, you are also getting water that way. Not to mention the many other nutrients your body needs to thrive and stay alive. But if you are consuming things that dehydrate your body—known as diuretics—such as coffee, alcohol, and very salty foods, then you need to drink more water.

A good general rule is to "earn" your other drinks by drinking sufficient pure, plain water. Want coffee in the morning? Fine. But sip on water before and after. And, yes, I said sip, not chug. Slowly replace that water you are using throughout the day. You should be drinking enough water that you are peeing about every 2-4 hours, and your pee is a light straw-colored yellow—not totally clear, nor bright or dark yellow. I cannot tell you how much just becoming more aware of your drinking habits and fluid intake can change your life. I have seen it every day in the clinic. Drink water! Be aware of what you put in your body, and how fast. Selfcare 101!

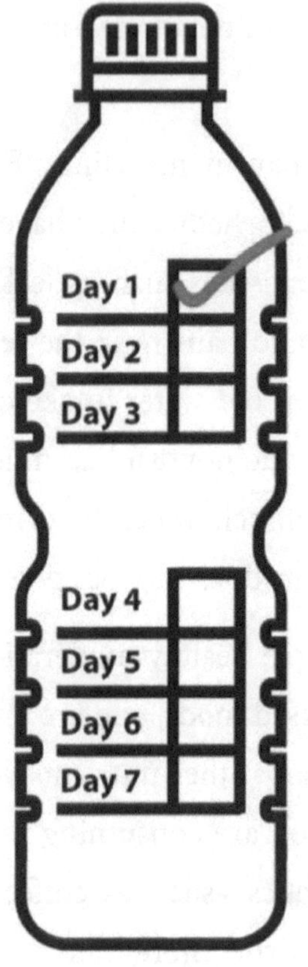

Daily Goals : _______

NEEDS BOX: IDEAS FOR BIOLOGICAL HEALTH RPACTICES:

Drink water for every cup of anything else, one-for-one.

Stop looking at all electronic devices for one hour before bed.

Go to sleep and wake up at the same time every night.

Eat the rainbow of colors in fruits and veggies.

Elevate your legs up your heart at night if you stand all day.

Do 10-30 minutes of exercise that increases your heart rate, makes you sweat, 3 times a week.

Keep up with you regular breast, gynecological, or prostate exams.

Use natural, healthy lotions for your skin and hair.

Use stress management techniques that work for you: breathe, journal.

Get a massage for tissue health once a week

Physical: What Does "Move and Groove" Mean for Me?

It is no secret that we are just not moving enough. Our lives are becoming more and more sedentary. We can blame many things; technology for one. The Selfcare Matrix is built upon empowerment and accountability. Look at how much you move in a day. Check your fitbit. According to the US census bureau, we are not moving as much as we used to. Our reasons or motivations to move vary from person to person. What motivates you does not necessarily motivate someone else.

SWEAT, STRENGTHEN, STRETCH: Why, How Much and What?

Many of my patients tell me that they are very active because they clean their house every day or are busy with household tasks, which is great. Housework does get you moving, bending, and reaching, which does bring blood flow to your tissues. That makes your tissues happy. It makes you happy to keep busy and have a clean house. But it does not promote balanced physical health. I also have patients who work out every day, often doing the same things; running and boot camp for example. This is not balanced either. Getting your heart rate up and balancing muscle length with muscle strength is what you should strive for.

You must find what motivates you. What type of movement makes you happy? I do believe the phrase "what you hate, you often need the most" can sometimes apply to food and exercise. But when you are just starting out with an exercise plan, choose what you like.

I hate running, but it makes me feel so amazing after I am done. I can no longer tolerate running, so I dance. Free form, dance-like-nobody's-watching kind of dancing. And on the days where I do not have energy to spare, I do easy yoga. For some, going to a gym, using a workout buddy, hiring a personal trainer, or finding videos is what works for them. How much and how often you move and groove will depend on your goals. Are you doing it to prevent weight gain, manage stress, or lose weight? Either way, I only ask that you follow these simple rules.

1. Cardio: Move enough to get your heart rate up as is safe for you. Check in with your healthcare team. Understanding what your target heart rate should be to achieve your goals is important. Here is one site that can help:

https://www.active.com/fitness/calculators/heartrate

2. Strength: Working on strength shortens the tissues; squats and lunges work on shortening the hip and leg muscles. Balance your movements to include all your joints, arms, trunk, hips, and legs. Don't just focus on your butt or abs. And know the difference between muscle soreness and joint pain. Muscle soreness ok, joint pain is not. (Think sore after running—OK—jumping off of a bridge sore—NOT OK)

3. Stretch: If all you ever do is shorten tissues, what do you think can happen? Our tissues are meant to shorten and lengthen throughout the day. This pumps healthy stuff in, and waste out, which is why repetitive use injuries happen. We do the same movements repeatedly without giving those tissues permission to move in the opposite direction, we get sore, the body protects itself, trouble occurs. If you lunge and squat, be sure to stretch the muscles you used before going about your day. If you sit on your butt all day, stretch your neck, back, hips and trunk, people! And remember, stretches feel uncomfortable but should not hurt after you are done.

4. Breathe. We have a tendency to hold our breath when we are concentrating, learning something new or when we are uncomfortable. Breathing while exercising is super important. Don't hold your breath! I promise you, you do it. At some point throughout your day you hold your breath. I hear it every day: "I had no idea!" Become aware of this habit and make a vow to change it. One moment at a time.

Here are a few examples of easy stretches and strengthening exercises that we all could use every day based on what daily life tends to require (Listen to your Body Here! If you are not sure; another question to add to your health care team list!)

Try This: Stretch a little…

Overhead Swiss Ball Wall Walk Arm and Trunk Stretch

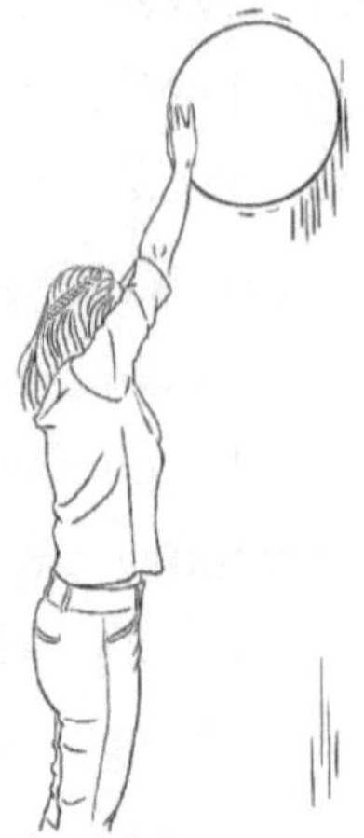

Standing Lateral Trunk Stretch/Doorway Stretch

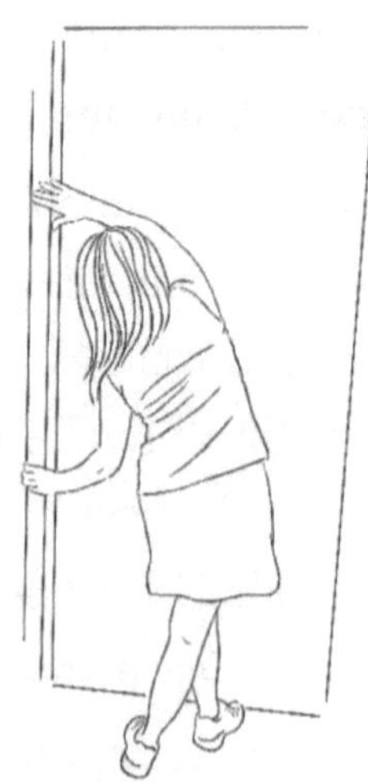

Seated Hamstring Stretch (30 second holds 3 times)

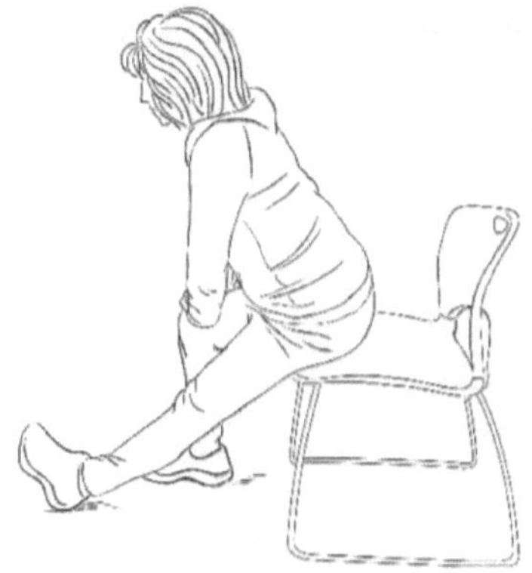

Seated Buttocks Stretch (only continue if pain free before and after exercise)

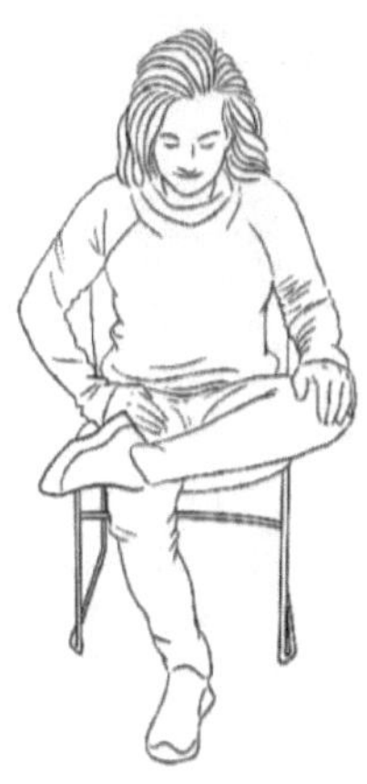

Beginner Leg and Core Strength: sink squat

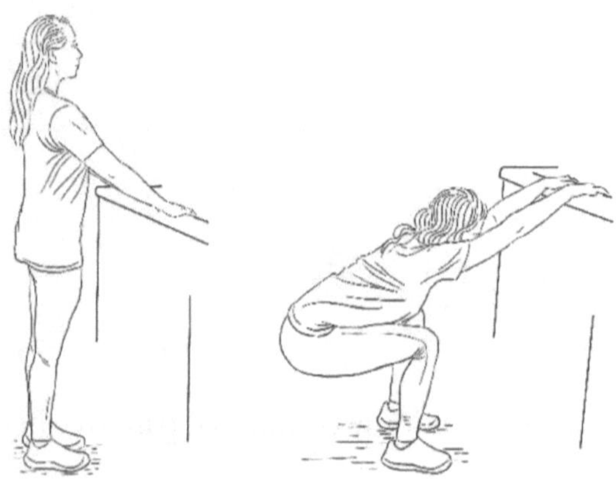

Leg and Core Strength: sit back (build up to tolerance, no jumping at first, or at all)

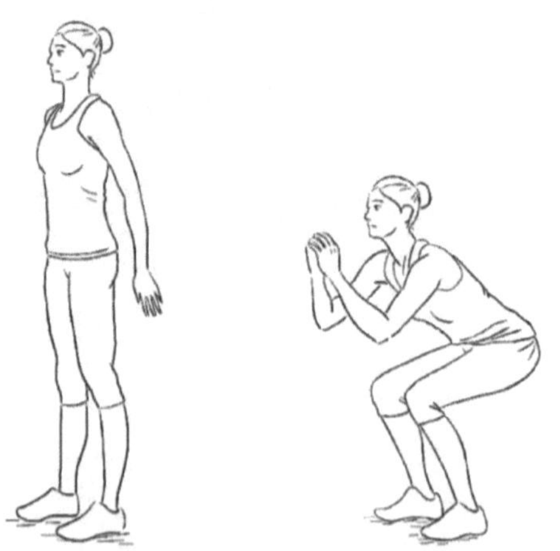

Leg and Core Strength: seated leg raise- pain free end range

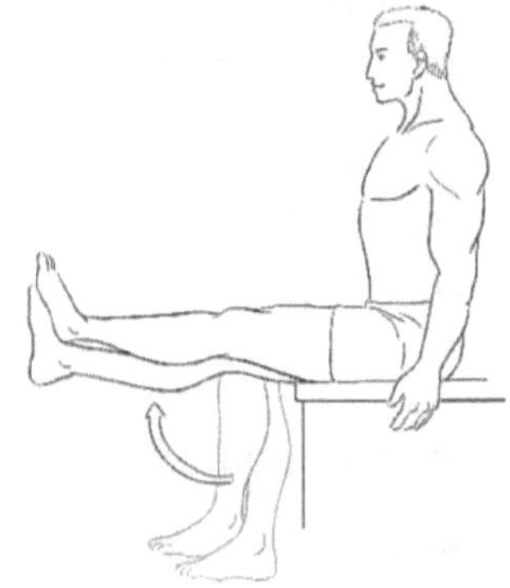

Hip and Pelvis Strength: Side lying **inner thigh** strengthening (life to comfort 5-10 second holds to rep tolerance)

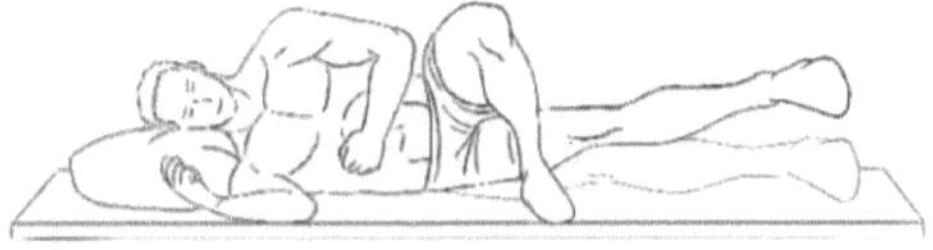

Hip and Pelvis Strength: Side lying **outer thigh** strengthening (life to comfort 5-10 second holds to rep tolerance, try not to rock your hips backward)

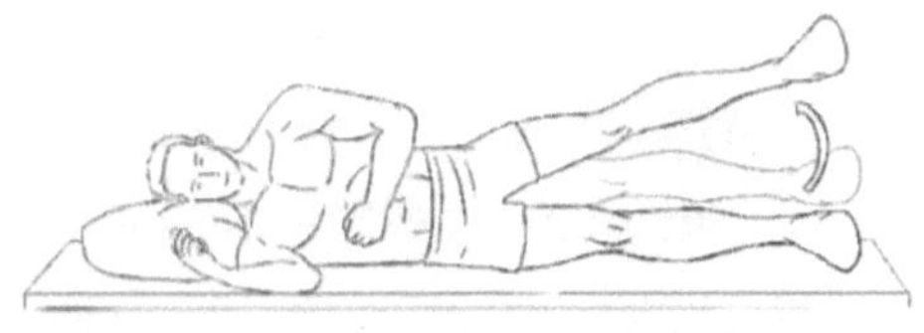

See Them in Action on Motivate Therapy's Youtube Channel

Sink Squat: https://www.youtube.com/watch?v=gOUR6RyskwE

BOX OF IDEAS FOR PHYSICAL HEALTH PRACTICES:

1. Do a few quick stretches with coordinated breathing before you get out of bed each morning.

2. Walk with a friend, neighbor, spouse.

3. Jump rope while watching your kids play.

4. Play hide-and-go-seek with your grandkids.

5. Learn ballroom dancing.

6. Take a free class to try: yoga, pilates, karate.

7. Swim or take a water class.

8. Find a personal trainer

9. Join a gym or class

10. Lie on the floor and stretch or foam roll while your family watches TV.

11. Train for a 5k, marathon, etc...

Mental: Why Just Breathe?

Have I mentioned how important breathing is for your whole-body health yet? Have you heard the phrase, "Take time to stop and smell the roses? Well, I believe that was code for "take time throughout your day and just breathe." Stop doing whatever it is you are doing, and just breathe. Earlier, I asked you to score, on a scale of 0 to 10, how you felt in your body. Take a few deep breaths and then check back in. What you were doing was what I like to call "getting out of your head and into your body" or giving the chattering "monkey" in your mind a banana. Telling that voice in your head to shut up and focus on something else, like breathing. If your score changed after focused breathing, then you effectively changed your mental state. And, as I stated earlier, if you change your mental state, you change the state of all six systems.

SILENCE and SIGH: Why, How Much and What?

There have been studies to show how diaphragmatic breathing improves many things in the body, including all eleven biological systems. Studies with healthy and unhealthy individuals typically show improved results. One study titled *"The Effect of Diaphragmatic Breathing on Attention, Negative Affect and Stress in Healthy Adults,"* showed improved test scores in emotional, mental, and cognitive health after performing an eight-week breathing training course. Another study showed significantly improved, long-lasting results with a one-week diaphragmatic breathing program for post-traumatic stress victims of the 2004 South-East Asia tsunami. Overall, many studies show that focusing on the sensations of your breath and slowing it down to about four breaths per minute can improve everything from anxiety, unclear thinking, stress, and heart health to bringing about improved attention, cognitive/brain function, and memory.

I have seen the power of breathing in my own clinic. It can give patients their lives back. Patients who have a constant urge to pee feel as though their lives revolve around the next trip to the bathroom. This is no way to live. Their bladder is in control, and therefore, their quality of life is severely affected. Yet, teaching them how to stop the panic cycle can be helpful. Stopping to take slow, deep breaths calms the anxiety associated with the fear of making it to the bathroom in time. Every time this works, it breaks the panic cycle and gives them a sense of control. Now their entire world has changed. And it can work the same for pain. [39, 40]

There are good free apps for your phone to help guide your breathing practice such as: "Health Through Breath: Pranayama lite" YouTube link at Motivate Therapy channel: Diaphragmatic Breathing! https://youtu.be/L5bRe28fCQA

BOX OF IDEAS FOR MENTAL HEALTH PRACTICES:

1. Take a meditation class.

2. Take slow deep breathes at each stop light.

3. Practice gratitude at each pause in life; stop lights, in between meetings, before meals.

4. Read one chapter a day on a topic that you want to learn more about.

5. Practice brain games that you enjoy; Sudoku, crossword.

6. Exercise.

7. Sleep 7-8 hours a night.

8. Try to "shut down" 15 minutes a day, power nap, breathing, enjoy nature.

Emotional: Don't Worry, Be Happy; Is That Even Possible?

As you read earlier, adopting some type of breathing practice positively affects all your systems. I separate mental and emotional for the purposes of stressing the fact that you need to pay attention to the health of each, but they are not separate. In fact, there is a medical health care specialty dedicated toward the study of the mind-body system, called "psychoneuroimmunology." Practicing breathing, becoming aware of the state of your emotions—as well as what triggers them and how it affects your whole-body health—is the foundation of self-care.

SMILE and SIGH: Why, How Much and What?

Research has shown the link between emotional health and immune system health—after all, the latter helps fight off infection and keeps you healthy. The research has shown that people with happier or more positive attitudes while receiving the flu shot were less likely to catch the flu. People who had the greatest activity in the part of the brain associated with depression when asked to dwell on sad episodes in their lives had lower antibody levels, or depressed immune system, after a flu shot. Yet, those showing the greatest activity when recalling happy times had more antibodies after the flu shot.[41]

More importantly, understand that there is no such thing as a negative emotion. All emotions play a role in your life. Sighing when you're sad, angry, or frustrated can feel great. If you never felt fear or anger, imagine what would happen in a dark alley when your life—or the lives of those you love—is being threatened. You would not have the instinct to fight for your life. Yet, often at a young age, we are taught that certain emotions are not okay, and we learn to push them down.

Not allowing yourself to feel or express emotions when you feel anger or sadness, can negatively affect your overall health. In his book,

When the Body Says No: Understanding the Stress-Disease Connection, Dr. Gabor Mate also discusses how depression refers not only to prolonged denial of your feelings, but also the effects of what it does to your immune system and overall health; it depresses it. It pushes it down.

So, allowing yourself to feel happy and to acknowledge and allow yourself to feel every other emotion your body offers in the moment, are part of the Selfcare Matrix.

It can be anything from smiling to yourself before getting out of bed, spending 30 minutes quality time reading, just hanging out with your kids, or jumping rope. Write a list of everything that you can think of so that on busy days you have options just as accessible as on days when you are less busy. And then, have an outlet to deal with every other emotion. Learn to recognize when you are anxious, worried, sad, mad, or depressed. Keep a journal, call a friend, meditate, pray— but allow yourself to feel it, acknowledge it, and move on. Just sigh, let go, move on.

Dancing like nobody's watching makes me happy, so I try to do it at least three times a week. Doing it every day would be even better, but I know that is not a realistic goal. My husband and I have found that giving each other the "heads up" that we are in a bad mood -I'm feeling [angry, grumpy]—is good for both our states of health. It allows me to acknowledge it and then, hopefully, he knows to try and be more patient with me and guide me out of it, usually by just talking about our day. Alone time reading also helps me move through anger, sadness, and frustration.

Try this: Stressed Out Situations

> *List five things that stress you out.*

Try this: Happy Times

> *List five things that make you happy and choose one to do this week*

Try this: Counterbalance

> *Try doing one thing on the Happy Times list after you experience stress in the Situation list*

BOX OF IDEAS FOR EMOTIONAL HEALTH PRACTICES:

1. Cuddle with your kids.

2. Go to a comedy show or funny movie.

3. Say thank you out loud every day.

4. Hold your partners' hand more often.

5. Make eye contact when you talk.

6. Give undivided attention to whomever for 10 solid minutes.

7. Watch an emotional movie with a group of friends then go out after to talk about it.

8. Walk with a friend or neighbor.

9. Journal.

10. Doodle or color.

11. Walk through nature or garden.

Social: What is "The Smile Heard around the World?"

Did you know that your smile can predict how long you will live? Have you ever had a stranger smile at you and notice that it totally lifted your spirits? The power of smiling is quite amazing. So why not smile to yourself, especially when you do not feel like it? Waking up and smiling to yourself, before you can even peel your eyes open, is a much better way to start your day than the phrase that often goes through our heads such as, "I hate getting up early," or "this sucks." You get better at what you practice. Begin your day practicing smiling to yourself, Then, one time today commit a random act of kindness by smiling at a stranger; you never know whether you might just make their day. Then perhaps that will inspire more random acts of smiling. The smile that is heard around the world. How powerful is that?

SOCIALIZE and SMILE: Why, How Much and What?

The wider your smile, the better. A thirty-year study at UC Berkeley examined the smiles of students in an old yearbook and measured their well-being and success throughout their lives. By measuring the smiles in the photographs, the researchers were able to predict a) how fulfilling and long-lasting their marriages would be, b) how highly they would score on standardized tests of well-being and general happiness, and c) how inspiring they would be to others. The widest smilers consistently ranked highest in all of the above.[42] Whether or not you have a strong social system right now, there really is no excuse to not be socially connected by choosing small daily interactions such as smiling to yourself and others.

However, this might not be as easy as it used to be. Unfortunately, it is becoming easier to go throughout your day without even making eye contact, let alone talking to another human, whether on the phone or in person. I am sure you have heard it said that social media is killing our social skills. Human interaction has been shown time and time again to not only improve your health but is essential to it as well.

If you have watched the survival show *Naked and Afraid,* you might have noticed that when one of the two contestants has to leave the experience, the mental and physical health of the lone survivor declines rapidly. We need each other.

A Harvard Women's Health Watch article discussed several studies linking social health to overall health. **Social connections give us pleasure while positively affecting long-term health and are as important as lifestyle choices and good sleeping habits.** People who have strong and consistent social interactions within their community as well as friends and family, are happier and live longer. Just like diaphragmatic breathing, a sense of social connectedness can improve heart, gut, and immune health. Another nine-year study showed that people who were isolated and not socially connected tended to die earlier than those with strong social health did.[43, 44]

And of course, the quality of your relationship counts. If you are happy in your marriage, then you will typically be healthier in general. It goes for your health care team relationships, too. Being happy with your doctor, therapist, or dentist is extremely important and will determine the success of the relationship and ultimately the success of your self-care. If you do not feel connected with your healthcare providers, you need to do something about it. You are the only one who can create the kind of changes that you need. Pure and simple, talk. Talk to your friends, talk to your family, talk to your healthcare team. Socialize and smile.

BOX OF IDEAS FOR SOCIAL HEALTH PRACTICES:

1. Contact (talk to) someone you haven't talked to in a while.

2. Join a group, such as a book club.

3. Hold your partner's hand more often.

4. Make eye contact when you talk.

5. Give undivided attention to whomever for 10 solid minutes.

6. Keep a consistent lunch or coffee date.

7. Walk with a friend or neighbor.

8. Volunteer.

9. Approach someone who is alone at a business function.

Spiritual: How Do I Let It in And Let It Go?

For this book, spirit is what makes you tick; what makes you the only you there is. It is your inner fire; what drives you, motivates you, gives you hope. Sound familiar? We talked about this in the intro. The heart of you is the heart of the Selfcare Matrix.

SILENCE, SMILE, STRENGTHEN: Why, How Much and What?

If you do not have hope, your health and happiness can take a major nosedive. You will no longer care to be "in the driver's seat" of your own healthcare. We have all had those moments where we just give up and say, "I can't take it anymore." But it is your spirit that says, "I refuse to give up. I won't just lie here and take it."

Life is about that constant push and pull. It is flexibility. Your spirit sees every failure as the entire reason to keep going, to try harder. The catastrophe of life. This inner strength—your fight and drive—lies at

196

the heart of the success of your selfcare matrix. It is what will drive you to act and no longer accept being a passive member of your team, but rather the one who is large and in charge.

This is freedom. As Oprah said in her June 2018 article *What I Know for Sure*, "...Freedom offers you the opportunity to stir things up, to bring your light, break up the darkness. To make your mark. Contribute. Give. Knock down the negative. And build a world worthy of your highest good." Living by the Selfcare Matrix is to be free and light. You are then free to give back and be charitable. This keeps your fire lit.[45]

For you, spirituality might mean your religion. Your faith in your higher power drives you and gives you purpose. So, be consistent with your faith practice—whether it is going to church, reading, studying, praying, meditating, repeating affirmations, or deep breathing. Spending quiet time with a group of like-minded believers—your circle of trust group—or yourself, is to renew your spirit. Just like your car or computer, your spirit needs to be re-charged every day. Practicing faith and gratitude, love, and kindness to yourself will allow you to project this to others. This is an essential piece of the selfcare matrix.

Ever since I was diagnosed with Lyme disease two years ago, I have experienced everything from severe head and ear pain to difficulty thinking, walking, sleeping and eating. Yet I continue to work, write, and live. Do I have good, bad, and horrible days? Have I questioned the universe, "Why me?" Yes, of course. But I know tomorrow is another day, so I keep fighting and people comment all the time, "I don't know how you do it."

Spirit is the answer. I have faith in my power to heal and in my purpose on this earth. To be a mother, a wife, a friend, a mentor, and a guide for patients that many others do not know what to do with. Those roles drive me. And guilt can punch me in the face when I feel that I fail in those roles because of the fatigue or mind fog.

But, I get to choose whether to let that guilt eat me alive or teach me a lesson. You get to choose what to let in and what to let go of. What you hold onto or practice every day will define you. No matter how I feel or what kind of day I am having, I look up to the sky and say, "Thank you! It is great to be alive." I let in gratitude and let go of whatever was holding me down at that moment. Then I do it again and again.

Letting go is the hardest thing to do, but it is so incredibly freeing. The hardest thing to do is often the best for you—having faith and a positive attitude, being thankful, and smiling. Connecting with yourself and others should always trump blame and shame of self and others.

To me, the term "free spirit" evokes a picture of someone who is happy-go-lucky and free to love others because they love themselves. Love is what put you on this earth and love is what will carry you through this life. But it has to begin and end with you—the whole you, the true you. And only you know who that is. Therefore, your health is in your hands. Be gentle, loving, grateful, and forgiving. Smile, sigh, and enjoy the ride.

BOX OF IDEAS FOR SPIRITUAL HEALTH PRACTICES:

1. Read one chapter of a self-help type book per day.

2. Read one chapter of a book related to your faith.

3. Join a group related to your faith or spiritual practice.

4. Meditate or pray 10 minutes per day.

5. Say, "Thank you it's great to be alive" at least once every day.

6. Be grateful for mistakes and failures.

7. Forgive for no reason and expect nothing in return.

8. Commit a random act of kindness.

9. Volunteer.

10. Smile or engage with someone you have never met.

11. Make a list of things that you like about yourself. Read it at least one time a week.

12. Just breathe and be.

REFERENCES

1. "Bibliography of Theodore Roosevelt." Wikepedia. Retrieved from https://en.wikipedia.org/wiki/Theodore_Roosevelt

2. Sartorius, Norman. "The Meaning of Health and Its Promotion." National Center for Biotechnology Information, U.S. National Library of Education, 2006; 47(4): 662–664. https://www.ncbi.nlm.nih.gov/pmc/articles/PMC2080455/

3. Rankin, Lissa, MD. "The Difference Between Healing and Curing." Psychology Today; 2018, Sussex Publishers. https://www.psychologytoday.com/us/blog/owning-pink/201110/the-difference-between-healing-and-curing

4. "Define Self-care." Dictionary.com, Unabridged, Based on the Random House Unabridged Dictionary, Random House, Inc. 2018. Retrieved from https://en.wikipedia.org/wiki/Theodore_Roosevelt

5. "Self-care." Retrieved from wikepedia.org. Wikepedia Foundation. Accessed Aug. 2, 2018. Retrieved from *https://en.wikipedia.org/wiki/Self-care*

6. "Define Self-care." Oxford Dictionaries.com. Oxford University Press. 2018. Retrieved from https://en.oxforddictionaries.com/definition/self-care

7. O'Dell, Brandon. "The Difference Between a Reason and An Excuse." O'Dell Restaurant. Blog at Wordpress.com. Consulting. Posted on April 4, 2008, by friendthatcooks.

https://blog.bodellconsulting.com/2008/04/04/the-difference-between-a-reason-and-an-excuse/

8. Ferriss, Tim. "Why you should define your fears instead of your goals." Youtube.com. TedTalks. Published by TED, July 14, 2017. https://www.youtube.com/watch?v=5J6jAC6XxAI and podcast

9. Roby, Becky. "Empowered." Urbandictionary.com, 1999-2018 Urban Dictionary. https://www.urbandictionary.com/author.php?author=Becky%20Roby

10. Popkin, Barry, M., D'Anci, Kristen E., Rosenberg, Irwin H., "Water, Hydration and Health." Aug. 2010. https://www.ncbi.nlm.nih.gov/pmc/articles/PMC2908954/

11. By Editors. *"Extracellular Matrix Definition."* Biological Dictionary. Retrieved from https://biologydictionary.net/extracellular-matrix/

12. "NIH Analysis Shows Americans Are in Pain." National Institute of Health. U.S. Department of Health and Human Services. Tuesday, August 11, 2015. Retrieved from https://www.nih.gov/news-events/news-releases/nih-analysis-shows-americans-are-pain

13. "Age Changes in Organs, Tissues, and Cells." MedlinePlus, US National Library of Medicine, August 14, 2014. Retrieved from https://medlineplus.gov/ency/article/004012.htm

14. Sonnenberg, A., Koch, TR. "Epidemiology of Constipation in the US." Pubmed. January, 1989. https://www.ncbi.nlm.nih.gov/pubmed/2910654

15. *Schwarts, Robert D, MD. "Somato-Visceral Pain: Undiagnosed chest, abdominal, flank & groin pain." Piedmontpmr.com. 2017. https://piedmontpmr.com/chest-adominal-flank-groin-pain/

16. Zimmermann M. (1989). "The Somatovisceral Sensory System." In: Schmidt R.F., Thews G. (eds) Human Physiology. Springer, Berlin, Heidelberg. https://link.springer.com/chapter/10.1007/978-3-642-73831-9_9

17. Sato, A."Somatovisercal Reflexes." Manipulative Physiotherapy. 1995, Pubmed, National Center for Biotechnology Information, U.S. National Library of Medicine. https://www.ncbi.nlm.nih.gov/pubmed/8775021

18. Nummenmaa, Lauri; Glerean, Enrico; Hari, Riitta; and Hietanen, Jari K. Contributed by Riitta Hari, November 27, 2013. "Bodily Maps of Emotions." Pubmed. PNAS January 14, 2014. 111 (2) 646-651. https://doi.org/10.1073/pnas.1321664111

19. Raab, Diana, PHD, "Calming the Monkey Mind." Psychology Today, 2018, Sussex Publishers. September 13, 2017. https://www.psychologytoday.com/us/blog/the-empowerment-diary/201709/calming-the-monkey-mind

20. By Editors, *"Body Systems Definition."* Biology Dictionary.net. Retrieved from https://biologydictionary.net/body-systems/

21. "List of Systems of the Human Body." Wikepedia.com. Wikimedia Foundation, Inc. last updated July 30, 2018. Retrieved from https://en.wikipedia.org/wiki/List_of_systems_of_the_human_body

22. *Garfinkle, Joe. "7 Steps to Clear and Effective Communication." Garfinkle Executive Coaching.com. Copyright 2005-2018, Joel Garfinkle.

https://garfinkleexecutivecoaching.com/articles/improve-your-communication-skills/seven-steps-to-clear-and-effective-communication

23. Eurich, Tasha. "Increase your self-awareness with One Simple Fix." Youtube.com, TedX, December 19, 2017. https://www.youtube.com/watch?v=tGdsOXZpyWEYoutTube

24. *"Definition of Matrix,"* Merriam-Webster.com, August 15, 2018. Retrieved from https://www.merriam-webster.com/dictionary/matrix

25. Dweck, Carol S. "Mindset: The New Psychology of Success. "New York, Ballantine Books, 2008. E-Book.

26. Briceno, Eduardo. "The Power of Belief-Mindset and Success." Youtube.com, TedX, Nov. 18 2012. https://www.youtube.com/watch?v=pN34FNbOKXc

27. "Water is Essential to Our Overall Health." Education.seekingheatlh.com Retrieved from http://education.seekinghealth.com/water-is-essential-to-our-overall-health.

28. "The Water in You." Water.usgs.gov. U.S Department of the Interior. U.S. Geological Society. Site last modified July 23, 2018.

29. Garland, Eric L., PhD. "Pain Processing in the Human Nervous System: A Selective Review of Nociceptive and Biobehavioral Pathways." Primcare 2012 Sept., Published online 2012 July 24. https://www.ncbi.nlm.nih.gov/pmc/articles/PMC3438523/

30. Moseley, Lorimer. "Pain Really Is in the Mind, But Not in the Way You Think." The conversation.com. August 6, 2012.

Copyright 2010-2018, The Conversation US, Inc. http://theconversation.com/pain-really-is-in-the-mind-but-not-in-the-way-you-think-1151

31. Kozlowska, Kassia, MBBS, FRANZCP, PhD; Walker, Peter, BSc Psych, MPsychol; McLean, Loyola, MBBS, FRANZCP, PhD; and Carrive, Pascal, PhD. "Fear and the Defense Cascade: Clinical Implications and Management." Ncbi..nblm.nih..gov. Harvard Rev Psychiatry July 2015. Published online 2015 July 8. https://www.ncbi.nlm.nih.gov/pmc/articles/PMC4495877/

32. Asprey, Dave. "Be Unlimited—Dr. Mark Atkinson #472." Bulletproof Radio. March 6, 2018. Copyright 2018, Bulletproof 360, Inc. https://blog.bulletproof.com/mindfulness-exercises-productivity/

33. Komnimnos, Andrea, "Maslows Hierarchy of Needs." The Interaction Design Foundation. https://www.interaction-design.org/literature/article/maslow-s-hierarchy-of-needs.

34. "Integumentary System." AAAS Science NetLinks. Retrieved from http://sciencenetlinks.com/student-teacher-sheets/integumentary-system/

35. Kashdan, Todd, B. "Psychological Flexibility as a Fundamental Aspect of Health." Clinical Psychology Review, November 1, 2010. https://www.ncbi.nlm.nih.gov/pmc/articles/PMC2998793/

36. Batmanghelidj, Dr. F. "You're Not Sick You're Thirsty." Watercure.com. 2008, Global Health Solutions Inc. http://www.watercure.com/

37. Leech, Joe, M.S., "7 Science-Based Health Benefits of Drinking Enough Water." Healthline.com, June 4, 2017. https://www.healthline.com/nutrition/7-health-benefits-of-water#section7

38. Xiao-Ma, Zi-QiYue. Zing-Qing Gong, Hong Zhang, Nai-Yue Duan, Yu-Tong Shi, Gao-Xia Wei, You-Fa Li. "The Effect of Diaphragmatic Breathing on Attention, Negative Effects, and Stress in Healthy Adults." Ncbi.nlm.nih.gov. Front Psychology, 2017. https://www.ncbi.nlm.nih.gov/pmc/articles/PMC5455070/

39. Descilo T., Vedamurtachar A., Gerbarg P. L., Nagaraja D., Gangadhar B. N., Damodaran B., et al. (2010). "Effects of Yoga Breath Intervention Alone and in Combination with an Exposure Therapy for Post-Traumatic Stress Disorder and Depression in Survivors of the 2004 Southeast Asia Tsunami." Ncbi.nlh.nih.gov. Acta Psychiatry Scandal, April 12, 2010. https://www.ncbi.nlm.nih.gov/pubmed/19694633

40. Battacharya, Shaoni. *"Brain Study Links Negative Emotions and Lowered Immunity."* Newsscientist.com. newsscientist Ltd., Sept 2, 2003. https://www.newscientist.com/article/dn4116-brain-study-links-negative-emotions-and-lowered-immunity/

41. Savitz, Eric.Guest post written by Ron Gutman. *"The Untapped Power of Smiling."* Forbes.com, March 22, 2011. https://www.forbes.com/sites/ericsavitz/2011/03/22/the-untapped-power-of-smiling/#708e70b37a67

42. Berkman, Lisa F., Syme, Leonard. *"Social Networks, Host Resistance, and Mortality: A nine-year follow up of Alameda County Residents."* American Journal of Epidemiology, Vol. 109,

Issue 2. 1 Feb 1979. Johns Hopkins Bloomberg School of Public Health 2018.
https://academic.oup.com/aje/article/109/2/186/74197

43. *"The Health Benefits of Strong Relationships."* Harvard Women's Health Watch, Dec. 2010. Retrieved from https://www.health.harvard.edu/newsletter_article/the-health-benefits-of-strong-relationships

44. Winfrey, Oprah. *"What Oprah knows for sure about finding hope and peace."* Oprah.com, Harpo Productions Inc. 5/15/18. http://www.oprah.com/inspiration/oprah-on-hope-and-peace

45. Worrell, Perri Dwyer, DC, DICCP. *"Why is chiropractic considered alternative medicine but physical therapy isn't?"* Quora.com, Jan. 23, 2015. https://www.quora.com/Why-is-chiropractic-considered-alternative-medicine-but-physical-therapy-isnt

46. Kearney, Gina, MSN, RN, CS, AHN-BC. Cioppa-Mosca, JeMe, PT, MBA. Peterson, Margaret GE, PhD. Mackenzie, C. Ronald, MD. *"Physical Therapy and Complimentary and Alternative Medicine: An Educational Tool for Enhancing Integration."* HSS J 2007. Published online 2007 July 28.U.S. National Library of Medicine national Institutes of Health.
https://www.ncbi.nlm.nih.gov/pmc/articles/PMC2504262/

47. Barry, Declan T., PhD, Beitel, Mark, PhD. Cutter, Christopher, PhD, Garnet, Brian, BA, Joshi, Dipa, BA, Schottenfield, Richard S., M.D. Rounsaville, Bruce J. M.D. *"Allopathic, Complementary and Alternative medical treatment utilization for pain among methadone-maintained patients.—An exploratory study."* AMJ

Addict 2009 Nov 16. U.S. National Library of Medicine national Institutes of Health.
https://www.ncbi.nlm.nih.gov/pmc/articles/PMC2777756/

48. "Sleep Deprivation and Deficiency." U.S. Department of Health and Human Services. Retrieved from Sleep Deprivation and Deficiency | National Heart, Lung, and Blood

49. *"How Does the Nervous System Work?"* Pub Med Health. National Center for Biotechnology Information. U.S. National Library of Medicine. August 19, 2016. Retrieved from https://www.ncbi.nlm.nih.gov/pubmedhealth/PMH0072574/

50. Courtney, Rosalba. *"The functions of breathing and its dysfunctions and their relationship to breathing therapy."* International journal of Osteopathic Medicine. Elsvier Inc. Sept. 2009, Vol 12.
https://www.journalofosteopathicmedicine.com/article/S1746-0689(09)00045-5/abstract

51. *"Your Digestive System and How it Works; What is the Digestive System?"* National Institute of Diabetes and Digestive and Kidney Diseases. U.S. Department of Health and Human Services. National Institutes of Health. Retrieved from
https://www.niddk.nih.gov/health-information/digestive-diseases/digestive-system-how-it-works

52. *"Bowel and Bladder Dysfunction."* John Hopkins Medicine. Health Library. Retrieved from
https://www.hopkinsmedicine.org/healthlibrary/conditions/kidney_and_urinary_system_disorders/bladder_and_bowel_dysfunction_134,113

53. *"Urinary System."* Innerbody.com. 1999. Retrieved from http://www.innerbody.com/image/urinov.html

54. Jones, Charlie "Tremendous," "Life is Tremendous: Do You Want to Be Happy, Productive, Healthy and Secure? Enthusiasm Makes a Difference." 1968, Executive Books.

55. Meyers, Thomas W. "Anatomy Trains: Myofascial Meridians for Manual Movement Therapists." P. 15, Churchill Livingstone Elsevier, third edition, 2014.

RECOMMENDED LEARNING RESOURCES:

Books:

- *"Mindset: The New Psychology of Success,"* Carol S. Dweck

- *"Full Catastrophe Living,"* Jon Kabot-Zinn

- *"Life Is Tremendous,"* Charlie "Tremendous" Jones

- *"A Guide for the Advanced Soul,"* Susan Hayword

- *"The Four Agreements: A Practical Guide to Personal Freedom (A Toltec Wisdom Book),"* Don Mig Miguel Ruiz

- *"The Coaching Habit. Say Less, Ask More, and Change the Way You Lead Forever,"* Michael Bungay Stanier

- *"How to Win Friends and Influence People,"* Dale Carnegie

- *"Yoga for Your Spiritual Muscles; A Complete Program to Strengthen Body and Spirit,"* by Rachel Schaeffer

- *"Why Pelvic Pain Hurts,"* Adrian Louw

- *"Explain Pain,"* David Butler, G. Lorimer Moseley (highly recommend the audio book)

- *"Yoga for Cancer: A Guide to Managing Side Effects, Boosting Immunity, and Improving Recovery for Cancer Survivors,"* Tari Prinster

- *"Anatomy and Physiology for Dummies,"* Erin Odya

- *"The Happiness Hack by How to Take Charge of Your Brain and Program More Happiness Into Your Life,"* Ellen Petry Leanse

Podcasts:

- *The Smallest Worthwhile Effect of Physiotherapy, Pain Science and Sensibility,* Sandy Hilton and Cory Blickenstaff, narrators. 035, Pt Podcast Network, August 17, 2018

- *Be Unlimited,* Dr. Mark Atkinson, narrator. March 6, 2018 Bulletproof Radio #472

YouTube:

- Ajayi, Luvvie, *"Get Comfortable with Being Uncomfortable,"* Dec. 1, 2017. TED talk.

  https://www.youtube.com/watch?v=QijH4UAqGD8&list=PLi4m29qWTtr39yTRN15Dg0usjOXejCxLx&index=8

- Eurich, Tasha, *"Increase your Self-Awareness with one Simple Fix,"* Jan. 11, 2017. TEDxMileHigh.

  https://www.youtube.com/watch?v=tGdsOXZpyWE

- Evans, Louise, *"Own Your Behaviors, Master Your Communication, Determine your Success,"* January 11, 2017. TEDxgenova.
  https://www.youtube.com/watch?v=4BZuWrdC-9Q

- *"Understanding Pain in Less Than 5 minutes, And What to Do about It,"* Jan. 15, 2013.

  https://www.youtube.com/watch?v=C_3phB93rvI

ABOUT THE AUTHOR

Denise is a wife to a wonderful, loving and patient husband. She is the mother to a son and a daughter who both love to read and write. They are her joy and her light. She loves nature, reading, hiking, cooking, and traveling. She admits—without shame—to being a geek on all levels about all things. She loves Sci-Fi and fantasy and any novel or text she can get her hands on; fiction and non-fiction alike. She is certified in yoga, massage therapy, pelvic floor therapy, biofeedback, and occupational therapy. She thanks her mother, father, and brother for instilling in her the love of learning, teaching, smiling, and laughing out loud a lot.

Your Selfcare Matrix

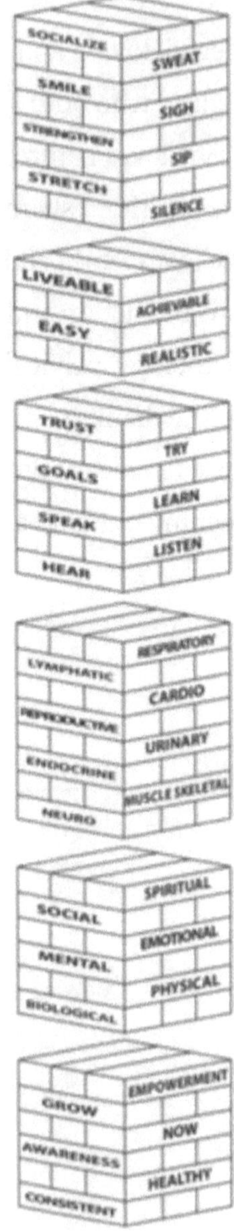

selfcare matrix

www.ingramcontent.com/pod-product-compliance
Lightning Source LLC
Chambersburg PA
CBHW051440250726
48655CB00001B/152